FAT TO SKINNY Fast and Easy!

Eat Great, Lose Weight, and
Lower Blood Sugar without Exercise

Doug Varrieur

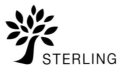

STERLING

New York / London
www.sterlingpublishing.com

The information provided in this book is for informational purposes only and is not intended as a substitute for advice from your physician or other health care professional or any information contained on or in any product label or packaging. The information and claims made in this book have not been evaluated by the United States Food and Drug Administration and are not approved to diagnose, treat, cure, or prevent disease. Check with your doctor before changing your diet. Author is not a trained medical professional. All references to manufacturer product information, labels, and web addresses are provided for informational purposes only and cannot be relied upon for accuracy as product information, labels, and web addresses change from time to time.

STERLING and the distinctive Sterling logo are registered trademarks of Sterling Publishing Co., Inc.

2 4 6 8 10 9 7 5 3 1

Published by Sterling Publishing Co., Inc.
387 Park Avenue South, New York, NY 10016
Originally published by Living Life Publications
P.O. Box 248, Maggie Valley, NC 28751
© 2008 by Doug Varrieur
Distributed in Canada by Sterling Publishing
c/o Canadian Manda Group, 165 Dufferin Street
Toronto, Ontario, Canada M6K 3H6
Distributed in the United Kingdom by GMC Distribution Services
Castle Place, 166 High Street, Lewes, East Sussex, England BN7 1XU
Distributed in Australia by Capricorn Link (Australia) Pty. Ltd.
P.O. Box 704, Windsor, NSW 2756, Australia

Sterling ISBN 978-1-4027-7133-0

For information about custom editions, special sales, premium and corporate purchases, please contact Sterling Special Sales Department at 800-805-5489 or specialsales@sterlingpublishing.com.

For more information, visit

www.FatToSkinny.com

This book is dedicated to all the

Special People

who simply want to be normal

HOW IT ALL BEGAN

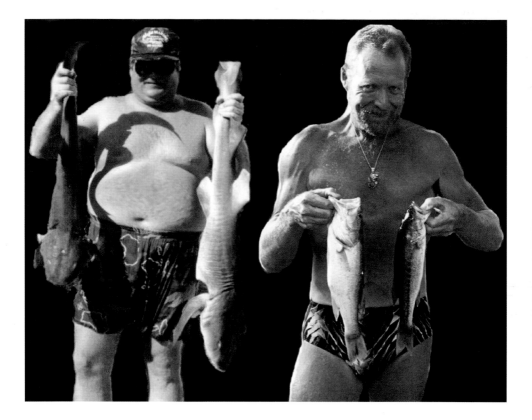

FAT TO SKINNY

Yes, this is me, in both photos. In the **FAT** picture I'm 35 years old and weigh 260 pounds. In the SKINNY picture I weigh 160 pounds and am 50 years old. At this point in my life, I've kept off the 100 pounds I **MELTED** off for the past 5 years. Want to know how? Read on!

CONTENTS

FOREWORD

Every day in my medical practice I confront obesity and its related complications. In fact these may be the biggest issues I face as a physician, for they can reach far beyond the waistline. Even mild obesity can cause imbalances in our bodies leading to high triglyceride counts, out of control cholesterol, insulin resistance, type 2 diabetes, and heart disease.

Obesity is an "equal opportunity" disease; it doesn't discriminate based on race, social status, income, or education. The truth is we are all susceptible to its onslaught. Doug Varrieur is a case in point. At the tender age of 12, Doug personified the fat kid, squeezing into size 38 jeans. By age 17 he had earned the nickname "Porky," and by middle age Doug had developed type 2 diabetes and suffered a near-fatal heart attack. At age 43, he made a conscious decision to make it his life's work to discover the answers to weight gain and weight loss. Luckily for us, he hit on a solution that not only changed his life but *can change yours, too.* Doug discovered that a single ingredient—*hidden sugar*—was responsible for his seemingly irreversible weight gain. After making this breakthrough, Doug lost 100 pounds, reversed his insulin resistance, and reversed his type 2 diabetes. Years later, he's still trim, healthy, energized, and raring to help others make the same life-changing discovery.

The result of Doug's seemingly never-ending passion for getting out the word resulted in this book. In *Fat to Skinny Fast and Easy* Doug tells his own inspiring story and gives us some startling facts about the ingredient we all hate to love and can't always see: sugar. For instance, did you know that a medium order of fast-food French fries metabolizes into the glucose equivalent of eating about 15 teaspoons of table sugar? Or that 2 cups of raisin bran results in as much blood sugar as eating 20 teaspoons of table sugar?

Doug has really demystified the processes that cause us to gain weight, and makes it easy to understand how to lose and then control weight, type 2 diabetes, and insulin resistance. His approach is so simple and clear anyone can follow his formula for success. The magic of his program is that it makes sense to everyone.

I've always thought that weight loss is very difficult and requires more discipline than most of us have. But after reading this book I think you will see it is really quite simple. And it's all backed by sound, scientific evidence. As a busy family physician I have long searched for a down-to-earth practical guide to losing weight. This book is that guide: whether you want to lose 10 pounds or 100 pounds it lays down the foundation for you and holds your hand on the journey to a healthier life. It empowers and educates you for a lifetime of healthy eating and living. For the first time in your life you will discover exactly why your weight has been a problem for you and what to do about it.

If you're a serial dieter who has jumped from one fad diet to the next—dropping pounds and clothing sizes only to watch your waistline balloon a few months later—Doug's simple, no-nonsense approach to losing weight and *keeping it off* represents real hope. If you can get hidden sugar out of your life you will not only get skinny "fast and easy" you will balance your blood sugar and reclaim your health and good spirits—without sacrificing great food or spending all your time at the gym. On Doug's eating plan you won't go hungry or feel deprived (the usual causes for falling off the wagon). Take a look at some of the delicious recipes and meal plans at the back of the book and say good-bye to the diet-starvation blues.

You've taken the first step by picking up this book. I'm sure you, like many of us, have tried diet after diet with little or no long-term success. The fact that you're holding this book in your hands tells me you have the desire to make changes in your life to lose weight and improve your health. Your desire, coupled with the power of this book, will give you the formula for life long success.

The key to weight loss and a healthier you begins with unveiling the truth about the ingredients that actually create fat and pack on pounds. In the pages that follow you will clearly see what those ingredients are, how to avoid them, and how to replace them with healthy alternatives.

Human nature dictates that most people simply don't care how much you know until they know how much you care. I can attest to how much Doug Varrieur cares. If there was ever a man on a mission to help you lose weight and regain your health it's this man. You will go from FAT TO SKINNY, and best of all you will do it with help from a friend, someone who has "been there, done that." Doug Varrieur is not only my patient, he is also an inspiration to everyone with whom he comes into contact. I can't emphasize enough what a service to society Doug has done by writing this book. I urge you to read it and follow the plan, for you too can go from *FAT TO SKINNY Fast and Easy!*

David Grant Mulholland, MD
Waynesville, North Carolina

IN THE BEGINNING

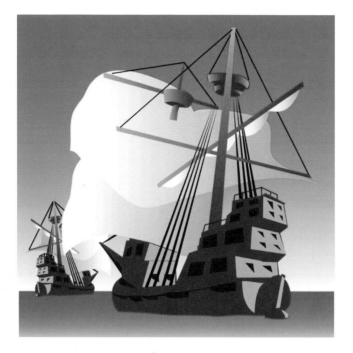

It all started with Columbus. You remember Columbus—everyone does. Columbus landed in the New World in 1492 and started the *maize craze*. Corn (maize) was a mainstay for the local Indians, and it wasn't long before this high-SUGAR, sweet tasting vegetable was a big part of the diets of the colonists who followed. It was easy to grow and had lots of uses. Corn was used as a fresh vegetable, and as ground meal for bread, soups, puddings, and fried cakes. Corn was also used as currency by the settlers to trade for other essentials. The colonists also fed corn to their livestock to *FATTEN* them up. As a matter of fact, we're still feeding corn to our modern day livestock to *FATTEN* them up.

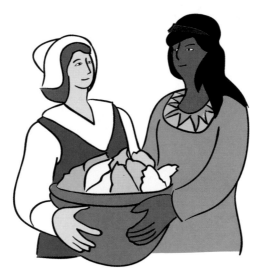

Columbus brought corn back to Spain, where it soon became an important food source across Europe. In 1493, Columbus brought a gift with him from the Canary Islands to the New World: *sugarcane*. Like corn, sugarcane also grows in tall, green, straight stalks. Once cut, the colonists would process it into SUGAR, which they used to sweeten their foods and beverages. They would then feed the pulp remains, along with corn, to their livestock. This was the beginning of the great American sweet tooth.

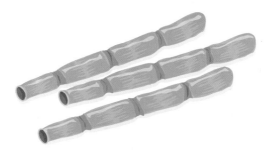

475 YEARS LATER

It was 1968, the country was heading into the Vietnam War, the Beatles had just released "Yellow Submarine," and Apollo 8 began its first mission to the moon. I was 12 years old. Mom and I were at our local downtown clothing store. (This was before shopping malls were popular and small towns actually had downtown retail districts.) The store was called Joubert's and it was the town's only full-service clothing store. By full-service I mean the store catered to all sorts of folks' clothing needs, including the *special needs people.* There's a certain connotation to that label, *special needs people,* and at the tender age of 12, I was about to find out what it was.

After the tape measure and the calculations were complete, this was the day Mr. Joubert announced to Mom that I was a *special needs person.* Of course, at that age, I thought that was pretty cool. It was like being a part of an exclusive club…the Special Needs Club. My only question was, *What am I going to get for a prize?* I didn't have to wait long for my reward; it arrived in the form of a pair of **Husky** jeans. Special jeans for *special people…Husky jeans.* There weren't very many varieties of these special jeans available at Joubert's clothing store; I had a choice between blue or black. Mom bought both. On the way home, Mom explained to me that I was a husky guy, AKA a big-boned guy, and the *special* clothes for the *special* people cost more money, so I should take particular care of them. I guess she didn't trust my jean-care judgment, because as soon as we got home she ironed a set of leather knee patches onto my new husky jeans in preparation for my boyish abuse. In her wisdom, she decided I would ignore her advice and be as tough on my new huskies as I had always been on all my clothes. Of course, she was right, and before you could say husky, husky, husky, Mom had transformed my new Joubert's special person's pants right into something out of an old western. Unfortunately for me, it was just one more thing that made me different from the rest of the kids. At least I didn't have to wear kilts, like my younger brother David did. That's me on the left with my 2 brothers, David in the middle and Donald on the right.

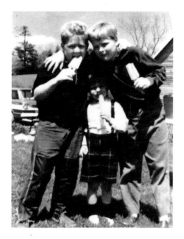

You're looking at a bona fide *special* person wearing bona fide *special* husky jeans while stuffing ice cream pops into his mouth.

Now, don't get me wrong—I knew I was fatter than the rest of the kids on my block. I was always the last one to get chosen for the backyard sports games, and wearing the most popular bathing suit of the day (Speedo) was completely out of the question. Mom always explained my size to me as being big-boned. "You'll grow out of it," she would tell me as she settled me down with…yes, you guessed it . . . food.

I'm not blaming Mom for anything, so don't misunderstand. Nutrition technology wasn't up to speed in those days, and most parents relied on the government's published food pyramid then as they do now as a baseline for their families' meal plans. Fast food really wasn't a part of the problem, because those types of restaurants were few and far between in our neck of the woods.

Over the next year, I grew, but I didn't grow out of "it" as Mom predicted, and I certainly wasn't in any shape to wear a *Speedo*. Instead, I grew out of my clothes as my waistline increased. By the time I was 13, I had ballooned to a size 38 pant. Mr. Joubert loved me—it was time for new huskies! That may not seem big by today's standards, but back when I was a kid. Childhood obesity was far less common than it is today. I was the **FAT** kid, and that was that.

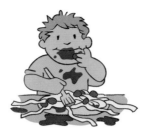

So there I was, the **FAT** kid, curly red hair, freckles, and with ridiculous patches on all my *special* pants. To make matters worse, I had to wear the wire headgear to straighten out my crooked teeth. All of this during school hours! YUCK! I'm amazed I survived childhood. There was no place for me in the social circles or on the school's sports teams. You know: *Fatty, fatty 2 by 4, couldn't fit through the bathroom door*. Kids are cruel. I don't think most kids mean to be cruel; I think they mean to be popular, or cool. Cruelty is simply the byproduct. That is, until—as most kids do—I found my niche.

The Boy Scouts of America became my social circle (they know how to treat the *special* kids) and I prospered within that micro-society for the next couple of years. By age 15 I was sporting a 40-inch orb and, like lots of kids, struggling with teenage acne. The difference was I was the **FAT**, curly redheaded kid battling my new physical flaw: zits! At this point in my life, girls had not even been an interest, and considering them was out of the question. After all, who wants to go out with the pimply-faced **FAT** kid? No one I knew. Girls were, however, the initial motivation for this *special* big-boned kid to attempt his first diet. Girls and *Speedo* bathing suits.

I made an appointment to go to our family practitioner, Dr. MacEnroe. Dr. Mac was a no-nonsense doctor who seemed to always have an answer for everything bottled up in a syringe, so I was a tad nervous when I arrived at his office. Needles had always made me squeamish, and I was sure I was going to be stuck with one from his funny-looking black doctor's bag. Not the case, however; no needles that day. Instead, the good doctor told me I was in excess of 50 pounds overweight, and he prescribed me diet pills to curb my appetite and gave me a pre-printed diet plan to follow. He then sent me on my way with a watermelon lollypop in my mouth. And so it began, the dreaded diet. Even though it was 35 years ago, I remember it like it was yesterday. It all began with a helping of a diet pill followed by this eating plan:

Breakfast…Black coffee, dry toast, and 1 half grapefruit with no SUGAR on top.

Lunch…Water or juice, small green salad, scoop of tuna fish salad mixed with cottage cheese vs. mayo, and a package of saltines.

Dinner…Water or black coffee, 6 oz of meat or poultry or fish, small salad, and a piece of fruit.

The next day came, and it all began again and again and again! Some of you may remember the diet, or some variation of it. Of course, the problem with that diet is the difficulty of staying on it for any length of time due to its lack of variety and flavor. And let's not forget to mention the fact that the curly-headed **FAT** kid was walking around *speeding* his brains out from the diet pills! So, like many diets that followed, it failed, and I continued to struggle with my weight. What made matters worse was that my chosen profession was to be a cook. Talk about giving an addict an unlimited supply of food fix!

By age 17 I had fallen into my identity as the **FAT** guy and had adopted the nickname "Porky." This emblem was mine until I left high school.

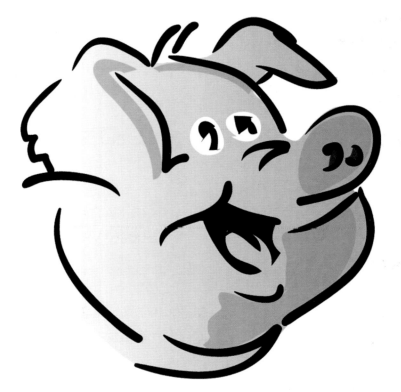

MY FIRST SUCCESS STORY

After I left high school, I took off and found my way to Texas. Having very little money and working 2 jobs, eating became a hit-and-run ordeal. I was busy, very busy, and I was motivated. My thoughts turned to straightening out my life and the food *issue* took a back seat. I ate less because I was running all the time. When I did eat, it was on the run, so I needed on-the-run food. I ate beef jerky, hard-boiled eggs, fruit, nuts, and veggies (such as celery sticks and bagged salads).

I was still living from paycheck to paycheck and restaurants were expensive, so I counted on a quick run into the local grocery store for food. When I wanted meat, I'd buy a small package of ham or turkey and a small block of cheese. Water was the beverage of the day because it was free. A simple stop at any public rest room filled my water bottle. This **FAT** guy found himself dropping weight like crazy and over the course of 6 months went from a 40-inch waist to a 32-inch waist. The first time I had ever been thin in my life! How simple…something else became more important to me than food! Without even realizing it, I had found a key, a key that I would later lose and not find again for over 25 years.

On my 18th birthday I called my mom to tell her about my weight loss and to bring her up to date on my life. I was proud to tell her I was no longer a *special person* at Joubert's and that I wasn't big-boned! Unfortunately, in my conversation with Mom, it became clear that I had to return home to handle some personal unfinished business that I should have handled before I left. It was time to say good-bye to Texas and head home.

Three weeks later, less than a year since I had left home, I arrived back in the little town of Whitman, MA. The **FAT** guy who had left returned home as the SKINNY guy. When I left, I had a big, bushy red afro, a 40-inch waist, and wore an army jacket with PORKY painted across the back. When I arrived home I was a 32-inch waist, had a clean haircut, and wore a suit and black patent leather shoes!

It was a glorious time for me. I settled into home life again and enjoyed living as a thin person for the first time in my life. Too bad it was short-lived.

MY FIRST FAILURE

In the first year after my homecoming, I went right back into the same eating habits I'd had prior to leaving. American Chop Suey was one of my favorite meals that Mom conjured up. The recipe calls for a pound of elbow macaroni, a can of Campbell's tomato soup, a large chopped onion, and ground beef. After the pasta is cooked, it is combined with the cooked meat, cooked onions, and soup to create Mom's delicacy. I loved it and always finished off a couple of bowls. Of course, it's Italian (sort of), so bread was a requirement with the meal.

Breakfasts were always fun and included fried potatoes at every sitting.

Lunch was typical: fluffernutter sandwiches, chips, and soda. For those of you who don't know what a fluffernutter sandwich is, it has peanut butter on one side of the bread and marshmallow fluff on the other. We also had strawberry fluff to shake it up a bit. Another favorite sandwich was banana and peanut butter. Just like ELVIS! It didn't take long for the weight to start coming back on.

My favorite vegetable was…you guessed it…corn! I loved corn, any way it came. On the cob, niblets, creamed—any way I could get it. Peas took a close second, and many times both were on the plate. Bread was served at every meal and I drank whole milk every day. My favorite snack was simply a banana, with a jar of peanut butter and a spoon to put it on top. Breakfast cereals—such as Fruit Loops and Cap'n Crunch—were always an arm's length away.

By age 20 I was **FAT** again. I never pieced together the food choices with my dramatic weight loss; I simply forgot. Food was so unimportant to me while I was in Texas that I simply credited the weight loss to all the exercise I was getting during my day job (walking in the Texas heat from home to home knocking doors) and to my night job (walking from station to station in the Levi's factory). I credited the weight loss to the lack of big, scheduled meals. The ingredient list was simply not focused on.

So there I was again, **FAT**. Not quite as **FAT** as before, but **FAT** all the same. My waist had ballooned back to a 38, and I struggled to keep it there. This struggle went on for the next 25 years. By age 30 I was bigger than ever. My waist was a size 44–46 and my weight hovered between 260 and 265. I was shopping in the Big and Tall stores and, once again, I had become a *special person.*

It was time to do something about it. It was time to focus on me. It was time to go on a serious diet. And so the battle began again…

THE **FAT**-FREE YEARS

Ah…the beginnings of yet another diet. This time I took the *fat-free* route. Fat-free products were all the rage, and I bought right into it. It was OK to eat potatoes—they're fat-free. It was OK to eat baked corn chips—they're fat-free. It was OK to eat peas and corn—they're fat-free. Fat-free salad dressings, fat-free mayonnaise, fat-free cheese, fat-free condiments, fat-free, fat-free, fat-free!

I lost weight. For me, the fat-free experience was responsible for the loss of about 30 pounds. Then… plateau. It didn't matter what I did; I couldn't drop another pound. For the next 13 years, the fat-free products helped my weight stay between 225 and 230 pounds. I had come to the realization that this was my "adult" weight, and if I could maintain it, I would be happy. I blamed it on metabolism, heritage, and age.

What I failed to blame it on was the one ingredient manufacturers of fat-free processed foods added back into their products. The ingredient to bring back the flavor they lost by removing the fat.

And then something magical happened.

FROM **FAT** to SKINNY AGAIN!

Mom and Dad live next door to me in the Florida Keys. They come down for 5 months every year and arrive sometime in December. Their arrival on the year of my 43rd birthday was different from all the years prior. This was the year my Mom and Dad arrived and Mom was thin! I've failed to mention to you that Mom has also struggled with her weight over the years, and at the age of 71 she managed to lose 40 pounds over a 6-month period. I couldn't believe it when I saw her upon their arrival. She looked 20 years younger and had the energy level of a 40 year-old.

When I asked her how she lost all the weight, she answered with 2 words: SUGAR CONTROL! I didn't have a clue what she was talking about, so we sat and talked. She had gotten herself involved in a low-SUGAR diet at the recommendation of her diabetes doctor. She explained to me some of the foods her doctor warned her to stay away from. A lot of it didn't make sense to me, so I hopped onto the computer and started to learn. The information I found astounded me, and I found myself experiencing that old feeling of hope. I allowed myself to consider that I could once again be thin, just like I was for a brief period 25 years earlier in Amarillo. Maybe I'd even get thin enough to wear a Speedo bathing suit. I got serious about SUGAR, and what happened next was nothing short of a miracle... that all boiled down to simple biology.

WHAT HAPPENS TO YOUR FOOD AFTER YOU EAT IT?

In my research, I found that regardless of what you eat, all food breaks down into one of 3 groups:

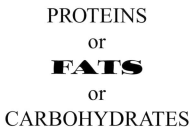

PROTEINS

or

FATS

or

CARBOHYDRATES

CARBOHYDRATES then turn into SUGAR.

What I'm about to tell you is not difficult to understand. I'm not going to go on and on, page after page, about the chemical process. Instead, I'm going to explain it simply because it *is* simple. So simple, in fact, that even to this day, years after I shed that last 60 pounds, the weight stays off! If you follow the rules I'm about to lay out for you and understand the chemical process in your body, you too will drop all the unwanted **FAT** that you want to—and you'll keep it off!

Are you ready for the key?

If you constantly battle your weight and seem to have a predisposition to gain **FAT**, then you're consuming too much hidden SUGAR! And like most of us who constantly battle our weight, you just don't know it. You're also well on your way to becoming *insulin resistant*, if you're not already there. We'll go into details about *insulin resistance* later in this book. The truth is, your weight gain and your inability to lose **FAT** is not your fault. (Unless, of course, you're a reader who is aware of your SUGAR intake and has ignored it. Then it *would* be your fault; you'd simply be lacking discipline, not knowledge.) I'll assume I'm surprising you right now and teaching you something you *don't* know. You're most likely addicted to SUGAR, like I am, and probably have been since a very young age.

Most overweight people crave and continue to eat foods they are addicted to day after day. We crave these foods because they make us *feel better* when we eat them. The average overweight or obese person has no idea that the daily food cravings and eating habits they are experiencing are the body's way of stopping *withdrawal symptoms* caused by the food addiction.

Why didn't Dr. Mac simply tell me I was addicted to SUGAR and high-SUGAR foods? The reason is that he—like most MDs and many other practitioners—simply wasn't aware of my addiction to SUGAR and its effects on my body. Only a specialist in this field would have been able to give me a diagnosis. Excess SUGAR and high-SUGAR foods in many people can—and does—cause weight gain and obesity, which in turn causes swelling, breathing problems, high blood pressure, heart danger, and in many cases, DEATH. The body's metabolic system simply can't keep up. The reaction to the body's inability to burn the daily intake of SUGAR results in excess **FAT**.

People's tolerance level to SUGAR will vary. In my case, I am a very active man, and still I am VERY sensitive to SUGAR in all forms. I gain weight very easily if my SUGAR intake exceeds 20 grams per day. Other people might not have such an intolerant disposition to SUGAR. Their metabolism may run more quickly than mine or yours, and they may be able to burn more of the high-glucose fuel with less effort. The easiest way to check your own tolerance is to remove SUGAR from your system altogether and start with a new baseline. That baseline will occur once you've attained your goal weight. At that point, you can experiment and start adding more SUGAR back into your system in measured amounts. These SUGARS will come in the form of *complex carbohydrates*.

SUGAR IS YOUR ENEMY!

SUGAR is what is making you **FAT**, and it's coming into your body from many different sources. Your body uses what it needs and then turns the rest into **FAT**. Once you know where all the SUGAR is coming from and understand what happens to it once it's in your body, you can start to make adjustments. Remember the gift of sugarcane from Columbus? It becomes *refined* SUGAR.

Refined SUGAR is found in processed foods, soda, candy, cookies, cake, ice cream, and any other products using it as an added ingredient. Refined SUGAR is a *simple carbohydrate*. The body burns it for fuel before it will burn anything else by immediately turning it into *glucose* (blood SUGAR).

SUGAR **from fruits**, *fructose,* is also a *simple carbohydrate.* Remember the body burns *simple carbohydrates* first for fuel before ever getting close to burning stored **FAT**. *Fructose* metabolizes slower because the liver converts it to *glycogen* prior to *glucose.*

SUGAR from vegetables and grains is a *complex carbohydrate* and burns more slowly than the simple carbohydrate. Although it burns more slowly, *in excess* complex carbohydrates will also cause **FAT** gain.

In excess happens more quickly with grains than with vegetables. Grains get turned into flour, flour gets turned into breads and pasta, and bread and pasta break back down to SUGAR in your body. (I bet you eat lots of bread and other flour products, such as pasta.) Grains also get turned into cereal, and cereal breaks back down to SUGAR in your body. (I'll bet you eat a lot of cereal. You may even put a high-SUGAR fruit on top along with a teaspoonful of table SUGAR.)

SUGAR is going into your system at an alarming rate. It's in your vegetables, fruits, processed foods, snacks, condiments, beverages, breads, and flour. Americans *live* on SUGAR. I mean that literally when I say it. SUGARS and added SUGARS are the main fuel of the American public! According to U.S. Department of Agriculture (USDA) data, SUGAR consumption in 1999 was 158 pounds per person! And SUGAR consumption is on the rise. In 1983, each of us ate 113 pounds of the stuff. Our consumption has risen every year but one since 1983. The USDA surveys indicate that the 158-pound figure is equivalent to around 50 teaspoons of SUGAR per day! What is the result of all this SUGAR? Over the last 20 years in the U.S., we have seen a 100 percent increase in obesity rates in children and adolescents. Added SUGARS include regular table SUGAR derived from sugarcane and SUGAR beets (sucrose), corn syrup, high-fructose corn syrup, corn SUGAR (glucose), honey, and others. These figures do not include the SUGARS in milk, high fructose fruits, grains, and high SUGAR content vegetables. All this SUGAR consumption over the years has created a vicious cycle for those of us addicted to SUGAR. The more SUGAR we eat, the more SUGAR we *crave*. Like the tobacco industry, it's the cravings that the SUGAR industry counts on to continue building its bottom-line profits.

So, now we know how much SUGAR we get from the SUGAR industry. How about the hidden SUGAR? This is the SUGAR coming into our bodies from high-SUGAR foods, such as fruits and vegetables. They come in the form of simple and complex carbohydrates. Four grams of carbohydrates metabolize the same as 4 grams of SUGAR. *To give you a visual, 4 grams of SUGAR equals 1 level teaspoon.*

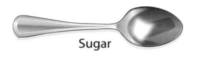

Sugar

So, how does our food compare to teaspoons of SUGAR? Let's analyze the SUGAR content in a medium order of fast-food French fries.

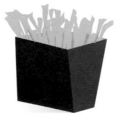

One of the purposes of your digestive tract is to break down the starch and other complex carbohydrates—which are simply chains of SUGAR molecules—into their component SUGARS so they can be absorbed into the blood. Our medium order of fries contains 47 grams of carbohydrates. Those 47 grams of carbohydrates metabolize the same as 47 grams of SUGAR, which is almost *12 teaspoons*! 12 teaspoons of SUGAR, just from the fries!

Now let's see what happens when we add a large soft drink, a hamburger bun, and a dessert:

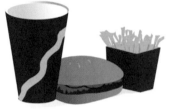 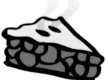

Sugar from fries	12 teaspoons
Sugar from soda	14 teaspoons
Sugar from bun	6 teaspoons
Sugar from peach pie	11 teaspoons

TOTAL SUGAR INTAKE: 43 teaspoons!

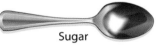
Sugar

Imagine what happens to the counts when we "supersize" our orders. No wonder the obesity and type 2 diabetes problems in the U.S. are running at epidemic levels. Eating this lunch is the equivalent of sitting down in front of your SUGAR bowl and eating **43 teaspoons of SUGAR—almost 1 full cup!**

1 CUP holds 48 teaspoons.

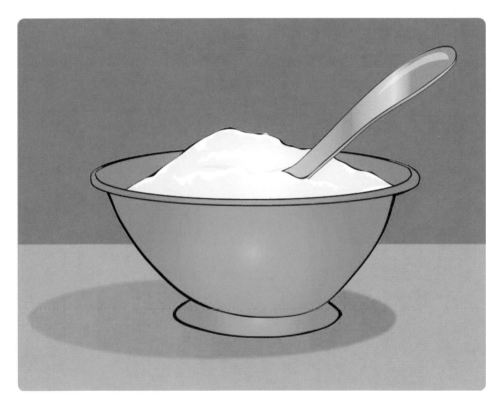

The only ingredient in the lunch that was SUGAR-free and good for you was the meat in the bun.

Now let's take a look at a typical breakfast.

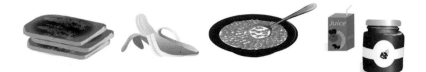

2 cups of corn flakes	**= 12 teaspoons of sugar**
1 normal size banana	**= 6 teaspoons of sugar**
2 pieces of toast	**= 8 teaspoons of sugar**
2 tablespoons of jelly	**= 7 teaspoons of sugar**
4 oz of milk on cereal	**= 1½ teaspoons of sugar**
6 oz box of orange juice	**= 5½ teaspoons of sugar**

TOTAL SUGAR INTAKE: 40 teaspoons!

Could you imagine how GROSS it would be to sit in front of your SUGAR bowl and eat 40 teaspoons of SUGAR?

Almost a full CUP of SUGAR

What about pizza? Pizza is one of our FAVORITE foods. There *can't* be any SUGAR in pizza…right?

Sorry! Let's take a look at a trip to the Pizza Parlor.

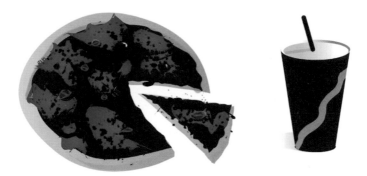

Pizza Hut 4-for-all Pizza Supreme

Whole pizza = **14½ teaspoons of** SUGAR

½ pizza for you = 7¼ teaspoons of SUGAR

24 oz soda = **19 teaspoons of** SUGAR

TOTAL SUGAR INTAKE: 26¼ teaspoons!

If you ate that breakfast, that lunch, and then a Pizza Hut dinner, it would be the equivalent of eating **109 teaspoons of SUGAR. That's over 2¼ CUPS! So much for a healthy day of American eating!**

Now you see the problem with the American diet, and probably *your* diet. The problem is that our bodies are not burning all the food we eat, let alone our excess **FAT**. Our bodies are burning the crazy amount of SUGAR in our foods. The result is, all the SUGAR that doesn't get burned turns into what? You guessed it ... more stored **FAT**!

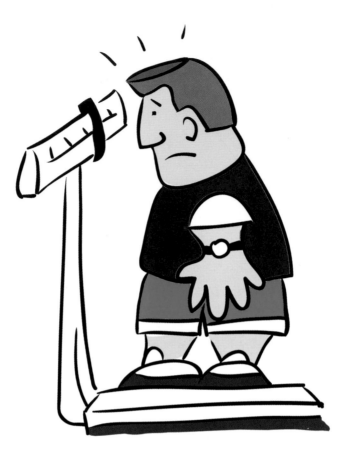

If you want to lose weight, your body needs to burn the stored SUGAR (**FAT**) for fuel. In order to get the body to do *that*, we simply have to cut off the SUGAR pipeline. This forces the body to attack those big, **FAT**, flabby deposits dangling around our bodies that make us the *special people* at Joubert's clothing store.

Cut off the SUGAR and you'll cut off the FAT. It's that simple.

So, how do we get rid of the SUGAR?

First we have to understand which foods in our diet are turning into SUGAR. Here's the answer: *all foods containing carbohydrates* turn into SUGAR… *gram for gram. 1 gram of carbohydrates = 1 gram of SUGAR. 4 grams of SUGAR = 1 teaspoon of SUGAR.* The body doesn't care what you eat or drink. It always breaks down the food or beverage into the same final ingredients. It doesn't matter whether the SUGAR begins as a complex carbohydrate SUGAR (found in flour and grains), a simple carbohydrate SUGAR (found in refined SUGAR additives), a fructose SUGAR (another simple carbohydrate SUGAR found in fruits), or a SUGAR derived from starch. All break down to the same thing— SUGAR—which in turn becomes glucose (blood SUGAR).

Carbohydrates In

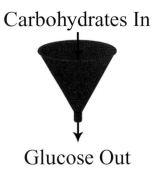

Glucose Out

Too much glucose, and BAM!! You get **FAT**, or worse, get **FAT** *and* develop **type 2 diabetes**. This disease is running rampant across our country, and you're at risk of developing it unless you curb the SUGAR. The following chart shows the SUGAR road.

All Roads Lead to SUGAR

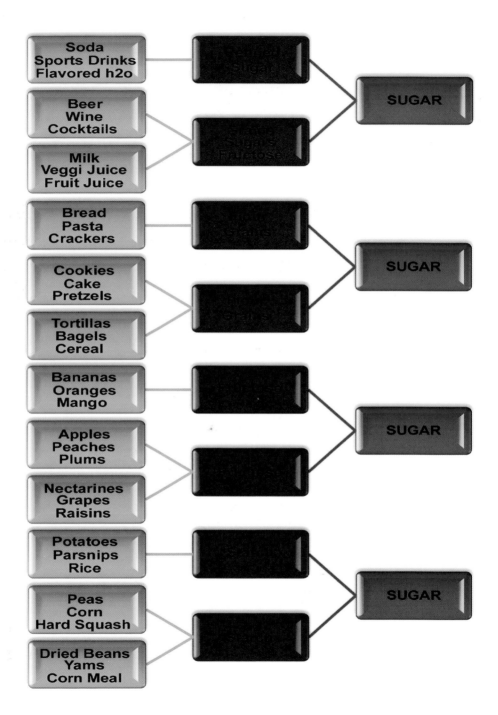

On the following pages I've outlined many common foods found in our diets. Next to each of the foods, I've broken down the SUGAR content in teaspoons. Take a look at this list and see how many of them are intermingled with your diet. Eating these foods gives you the same number of carbohydrates as if you were to eat the number of teaspoons of table SUGAR that I have listed beside each item.

From this point forward, I want you to *SEE* the hidden SUGARS in your food and imagine yourself sitting down at the SUGAR bowl with a teaspoon and eating pure SUGAR as you eat these foods. Then you'll see clearly the amount of SUGAR you consume daily.

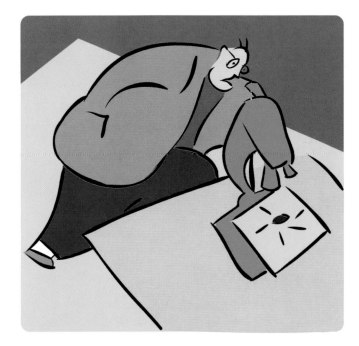

JUST A SPOONFUL OF SUGAR
How bad can it be?

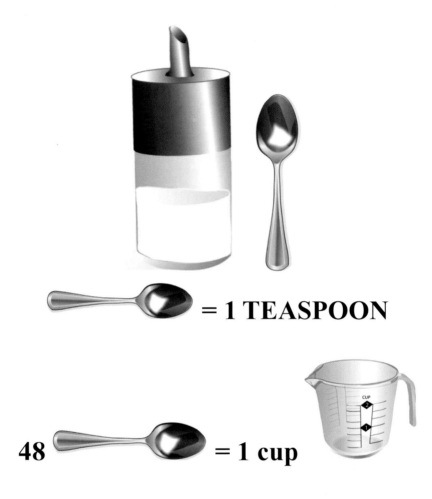

= 1 TEASPOON

48 = 1 cup

BEVERAGES

Soda (24 oz)	19	sugar
Orange juice (8 oz)	6½	sugar
Apple juice (8 oz)	7	sugar
Beer (12 oz)	3	sugar

Milk 2% (8 oz)	3	sugar
Pina Colada (3½ oz)	6	sugar
Margarita (3½ oz)	3½	sugar
Hot chocolate (8 oz)	8	sugar
Gatorade (8 oz)	4	sugar

BREAD

I've eaten bread with every meal my whole life! Bagels were always one of my favorites until I discovered eating my bagel was the equivalent of eating 8 teaspoons of SUGAR right from the SUGAR bowl!

Bagel (3½ in)	8	sugar
Cornbread (5-in square)	9	sugar
English muffin, plain	6	sugar
English muffin, raisin	6½	sugar
French bread (3 oz)	9	sugar
Italian bread (3 oz)	9	sugar
Oatmeal (3 oz)	8	sugar
Pita, white (7 in)	7½	sugar
Pita, wheat (7 in)	7½	sugar
Pumpernickel (3 oz)	7½	sugar
Raisin bread (3 oz)	9	sugar
Rye bread (3 oz)	7½	sugar
Sourdough bread (3 oz)	9	sugar
Tortillas, corn, small	2½	sugar

Tortillas, flour, small	5½	sugar
Tortillas, wheat, small	4	sugar
Tortilla, La Tortilla Factory	½	sugar
Wheat bread (3 oz)	7½	sugar
White bread (3 oz)	8½	sugar
Whole grain bread (3 oz)	8	sugar

CEREALS

All 1-cup measurements

(I don't know about yours, but my cereal bowls all hold more than 1 cup!)

Cheerios	3½	sugar
Cocoa Puffs	6½	sugar
Corn Chex	6	sugar
Corn Flakes	6	sugar
Cracklin' Oat Bran	10	sugar
Cream of Wheat	7	sugar
Crispix	6	sugar
Fiber One	5	sugar
Frosted Flakes	9	sugar
Frosted Mini-Wheats	10	sugar
Froot Loops	7	sugar
Grape-Nuts	7	sugar

Grits	8	sugar
Life	8	sugar
Nut & Honey Crunch	7½	sugar
Puffed Rice	3	sugar
Raisin Bran	10	sugar
Rice Krispies	5½	sugar
Shredded Wheat	5	sugar
Special K	5½	sugar
Wheaties	5	sugar

CRACKERS

Cheez-It (20)	3	sugar
Harvest Crisps (20)	8½	sugar
Ritz (10)	5	sugar
Saltines (6)	3	sugar
Town House (8)	4	sugar
Triscuit (6)	4	sugar
Wheat Thins (20)	6	sugar

DESSERTS

Brownie (1)	6	sugar
Yellow cake (1/12)	9	sugar
Apple pie (1/8)	10	sugar
Cherry pie (1/8)	12	sugar

Milky Way (1 bar)	10	sugar
Hershey's Kisses (10)	7	sugar
Snickers (2 oz bar)	8	sugar
Oatmeal cookie (2)	8	sugar
Fig bar (4)	10	sugar

FRUITS

Apple	3½	sugar
Apricot (3)	2	sugar
Avocado, Haas	1	sugar
Banana (small)	4½	sugar
Blackberries (½ cup)	1	sugar
Blueberries (½ cup)	2½	sugar
Grapefruit	4	sugar
Grapes (1 cup)	7	sugar
Mango (1 cup)	6	sugar
Melon (1 cup)	4	sugar
Orange	3	sugar
Peach	2½	sugar
Pear	5	sugar
Pineapple (1 cup)	5	sugar
Raisins (½ cup)	13	sugar
Raspberries (½ cup)	1	sugar
Strawberries (½ cup)	½	sugar

PASTA & RICE

Pasta (1½ cups)	15 sugar
Pasta, wheat (1½ cups)	13 sugar
Rice, white (1 cup)	11 sugar
Rice, brown (1 cup)	11 sugar

SNACKS

Cheetos (30)	5 sugar
Fritos (30)	3 sugar
Pringles (20)	5 sugar
Pretzels (35 sticks)	4 sugar
Tortilla chips (30)	7½ sugar

By now you should have a good understanding of where your SUGAR is coming from. As you read labels, you'll look for the carbohydrate counts in the food. That's the way the FDA requires the food manufacturers to report the SUGAR content in our foods. Remember the formula: Your body metabolizes every 4 grams of carbs the same as it would metabolize 1 teaspoon of SUGAR.

Remember the first diet I went on when I was fifteen? You know, the Dr. MacEnroe diet? Let's take a look at it again…this time we'll look at the numbers in terms of SUGAR content.

Breakfast…Black coffee, dry toast, and 1 half grapefruit, no SUGAR on top.

Lunch…Water or juice, small green salad, scoop of tuna fish salad mixed with cottage cheese vs. mayo, and a package of saltines.

Dinner…Water or black coffee, 6 oz of meat or poultry or fish, small salad, and a piece of fruit.

Let's examine Dr. MacEnroe's diet:

Black coffee	¼	sugar
Dry toast (2 pieces)	7	sugar
Half a grapefruit	4	sugar

Green salad	½	sugar
Tuna fish	0	sugar
Cottage cheese	½	sugar
Saltines (6)	3	sugar
Orange juice (8 oz)	5	sugar

Black coffee	¼	sugar
Meat (6 oz)	0	sugar
Green salad	½	sugar
Banana	4½	sugar

TOTAL SUGAR: 26 TEASPOONS! The equivalent of 104 carbohydrates. We have to remove the fiber content from the carbs to get a **net** carb count. The fiber content for the day was only 6 grams. That leaves **98 grams** of **net** carbohydrates for Dr. Mac's daily diet! That equates into 98 grams of SUGAR divided by 4, which equals 24½ teaspoons of SUGAR!

If you're **FAT** and want to burn **FAT**, you need to keep your total intake to no more than **5 teaspoons of SUGAR from all sources per day.**

That means your total carbohydrate intake must be no more than **20 grams of total net carbohydrates for the entire day**. If you want your body to search out the **FAT** and use it for fuel, cut off the SUGAR fuel source by mouth and that's exactly what will happen. Your body will seek out the SUGAR it needs from the storage areas around your body. You'll shrink like the incredible shrinking person! And you can do it without being hungry.

No wonder Dr. Mac's diet and others like it have failed people for so many years. It's loaded with hidden SUGAR! This is also the problem with fat-free programs. Flavor is lost in products when they remove the **FAT**, so the manufactures add another ingredient to make up for the flavor loss. Any guesses? I was amazed when I checked the labels. Most manufactures replace the **FAT** with…you guessed it…SUGAR! Again, the culprit in a **FAT**-free diet comes down to SUGAR.

I know what you're thinking. *He's taking away ALL my food. I have to starve myself.* Quite the contrary! If you follow this high-protein, low-SUGAR eating program, you'll never feel hungry. You'll eat wonderful food, and you will lose lots of **FAT** and keep it off! The trick is knowing what foods to eat, how to prepare them, and how to replace your favorite high-SUGAR foods with low-SUGAR foods.

I'm going to take all the guesswork out of it for you. As you continue to read on, you'll find I've outlined your new ingredient lists, given you favorite replacement recipes, and supplied you with web links and products to keep your variety exciting. I'm also going to give you information about my blood profile and explain to you the effects on triglycerides and cholesterol that result from this kind of eating plan. In short, I'm going to dedicate the rest of this book to *you and your success* in the quest to be SKINNY. Your job is to understand the methods and apply them. *Knowing* the information is only half the battle; *doing something* with the information is the other half. One is no good without the other.

What do you say? Are you ready to get started on a new and slender you? Are you ready to fit into those high school sizes again? Are you ready for your *miracle?*

Are You Ready to Slay the SUGAR Dragon?

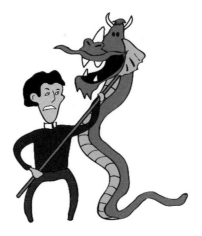

Let's Get Started!

First, we need to know how to read those labels. Let's take a look at this one. This is the pertinent information from the nutritional label for a 20-piece order of Chicken McNuggets from McDonald's:

NUTRITION FACTS
Serving size 20 pieces (320 grams)

Calories	840
Calories from Fat	441
Total Fat	49g
Saturated Fat	11g
Cholesterol	125mg
Sodium	2240mg
Total Carbohydrates	**51g**
Protein	50g

The ingredient you're looking for is
Total Carbohydrates   51 grams

51 grams divided by 4 equals 12¾ teaspoons of SUGAR. It will interest you to know that ALL of the SUGAR is coming from the coating on the chicken nuggets, and not from the chicken itself, nor from the oil used to cook it in.

The next product is chicken without a coating. Let's do another label. This one is the pertinent information from the nutritional label for frozen Tyson brand chicken breast strips. Let's look at the carb count in the chicken alone.

NUTRITION FACTS
Serving size 3 oz (84 grams)

Calories	120
Calories from Fat	32
Total Fat	3.5g
Saturated Fat	1g
Polyunsaturated Fat	.5g
Monounsaturated Fat	1.5g
Cholesterol	60mg
Sodium	500mg
Total Carbohydrates	**1g**
Protein	21g

Total Carbohydrates   1 gram

As you can see, the carb count in chicken without breading is VERY low. In this case, 1 gram per serving size, which is only ¼ teaspoon of SUGAR. That means you would have to eat 51 servings of this chicken to get the same amount of carbs into your body as you'll get from one 20-piece order of Chicken McNuggets!

Let's take a look at soda. This is a 14 oz mug of SUGAR-free A&W Root Beer. Here is the pertinent information from the nutritional label:

NUTRITION FACTS

Serving size 1 serving (397 grams)

Calories	0
Calories from Fat	0
Total Fat	0g
Sodium	35mg
Total Carbohydrates	**0g**
Protein	0g

Total Carbohydrates 0 grams

Below is another mug of root beer, 14 oz, and also A&W. Except, this mug is NOT SUGAR-free. This is the pertinent information from the nutritional label:

NUTRITION FACTS

Serving size 1 serving (397 grams)

Calories	190
Calories from Fat	0
Total Fat	0g
Sodium	35mg
Total Carbohydrates	**51g**
Sugars	**51g**
Protein	0g

Total Carbohydrates 51 grams

Look at the carbohydrate count: 51 grams. Now look at the SUGARS count. What do you see?…51 grams. Exactly the same as the carb count. The difference between the 2 sodas is the one that will make you **FAT** is the one that contains over 12 teaspoons of SUGAR (51 divided by 4 = 12¾). So what are we learning? It's ALL about choices. It's time to **LEARN YOUR FOOD!**

Now you know that an order of 20 Chicken McNuggets and a 14 oz mug of root beer contains over 63 teaspoons of SUGAR. You also now know that the same size serving of un-breaded chicken strips and a 14 oz mug of SUGAR-free root beer only contains ¼ teaspoon of SUGAR.

Which one are you going to eat? See, it's all about choices. Choose to eat products with VERY low carbohydrate counts on the labels and you'll lose **FAT**.

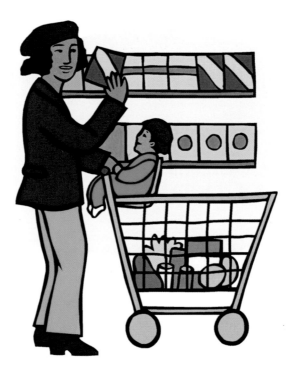

WHY DO I GET **FAT**?

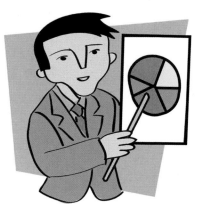

I know you're excited and more than ready to get this going, but we do need to touch on the science so you completely understand what is happening in your body. This is the stuff they should have taught us in grammar school! Let's start with proteins and fats. Both proteins and fats metabolize in your body slowly. They turn into fuel gradually, and they do not cause an *insulin reaction*. The only way you'll gain weight eating proteins and fats is by *over*eating proteins and fats.

Carbohydrates are completely different. Eating carbs does create an insulin reaction. It's that insulin reaction that causes weight gain. Here's the simple explanation: When you eat any high-glycemic (fancy word for SUGAR) foods high in carbs, the body turns it into *glucose, AKA blood SUGAR*, in your digestive tract. The glucose is then absorbed into your blood stream. The SUGAR entering your blood stream then causes the *pancreas* to pour insulin into the blood, creating an *insulin spike*. Insulin is the *gatekeeper* for your cells. Each of your cells is a little *furnace* waiting for fuel to burn, but the fuel can't get in without the gatekeeper opening the gate. The job of insulin is to go to the cells floating around in your blood and attach itself to each cell. Once the insulin attaches itself to your cells, it opens up the cell to allow the SUGAR to enter the furnace to be burned. The body will burn what it needs based on your activity level, and then the *liver* converts all of the unused SUGAR into short- and long-term energy stores. Short-term glycogen is stored in your liver and muscle tissue, while long-term **FAT** gets stored in your **FAT** cells.

If you're **FAT**, it's because more SUGAR is going *in* than is being burned. Your chances of burning off more of the blood SUGAR increases dramatically if your body is revved up from strenuous exercise *and* you eat no more SUGAR than will burn off while your body is in a metabolizing state from that exercise. For most **FAT** people, that is not the case, but let's talk about *you*. When you sit down to eat a meal, are you within a half hour of coming from hard exercise? Or are you sitting at your desk, driving in your car, or watching TV?

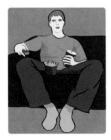

If you're like most of us **FAT** people, your body is sedentary when you eat and therefore has a less than fired-up metabolism. The furnaces in your cells are out. Your SUGAR intake is not getting burned; it's being stored for a rainy day inside your **FAT** cells. To make matters worse, you're probably into a bag of chips or snacks between meals, or worse, you ate a Big Mac in the car on the way home from work before dinner like I used to! All this SUGAR is causing insulin spikes.

It's the insulin spike that creates the problem. The insulin we produce in our bodies is our **FAT**-making hormone. Its job is to deal with the blood SUGAR by opening the furnace to allow it to be burned.

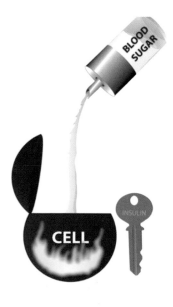

CELL
UNLOCKED BY INSULIN BURNING SUGAR

Once the body has burned all the fuel it needs, the fire in the furnace goes out. If you've taken in more SUGAR than the body needs, the liver will turn some of the excess glucose into glycogen for short-term energy stores, and the rest ends up in long-term storage as **FAT** to be reserved in your **FAT** cells.

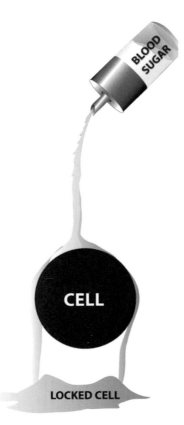

Locked Cell, Blood SUGAR Can't Get In

Fire's out, boys. Time to store the SUGAR!

Where do you guys want to stick it?

Let's put it in the **FAT** cells on the belly!

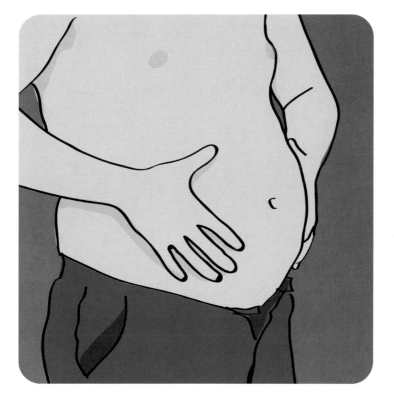

You can change this **Fast and Easy!**

HOW DO I LOSE **FAT**?

Losing **FAT** is as simple as gaining **FAT**. To lose **FAT**, keep the SUGAR intake low and the glucose levels will stay low. Keep the glucose levels low and the insulin levels will stay low. Keep the insulin levels low and the **FAT** production ceases. It's that simple! All you need to do is switch fuels from fast-burning fuels (carbohydrates) to slow-burning fuels (proteins and fats). Your body will do the rest. Because of the enormity of the obesity problem in our country and the propaganda the diet industry feeds our minds, most of us believe the answer to **FAT** loss must be more complicated than this, but it's not. Fuel is fuel, and the body will seek out the fuel it needs within the body structure if you deny it entry by mouth. You don't need diet pills, you don't need expensive exercise equipment, you don't need to buy elixirs, and you don't need costly, prepared diet food shipped to your door. You simply have to understand body fuel.

This is the order in which your body burns fuel:

1st to burn, fuel #1—*Carbohydrates*, which have turned into glucose (blood SUGAR).

2nd to burn, fuel #2—*Glycogen*, stored glucose in the liver and muscle tissue.

3rd to burn, fuel #3—**FAT** *stores* in your body stored in **FAT** cells. The **FAT** you want to lose.

4th to burn, fuel #4—*Protein*, used to replenish body tissue. Any excess will be burned as fuel.

To get your body to the point where it starts burning your **FAT** stores, remove fuel #1, deplete fuel #2, and watch the magic begin.

To get your body to gain **FAT**, give it more SUGAR than can be burned during the corresponding insulin spike from eating excess fuel #1, and BINGO! You'll gain **FAT**. To get your body to stay the same weight and neither lose **FAT** nor gain **FAT**, only take in as much SUGAR from fuel #1 as you can burn during a particular activity. If all the SUGAR gets burned in the cells, you'll neither gain nor lose weight. It's all about scheduling your SUGAR intake based on:

Whether you want to lose **FAT**.

Whether you want to gain **FAT**.

Whether you want to stay the same weight.

Your goal should be to lose all the **FAT** you want until you get to the size you want to be. Once you're at your goal size, you'll want to maintain that size and not fluctuate more than 5 pounds either way for the rest of your life. You can maintain your new weight very simply by scheduling your food intake based on your activity level.

THIS IS NOT A DIET

This program is not a diet; it's the furthest thing from a diet. Diets don't work. The very thought of a diet leads us to the understanding that it is temporary. This eating plan is not temporary. This eating plan is an identification process of the one ingredient that has made you **FAT** and kept you **FAT**: SUGAR.

This is an opportunity that will train you to remove SUGAR from your everyday food intake, allowing you to live your life as a healthy, vibrant SKINNY person never fighting the weight battle again.

Knowledge is your hammer; SUGAR removal is your winning blow.

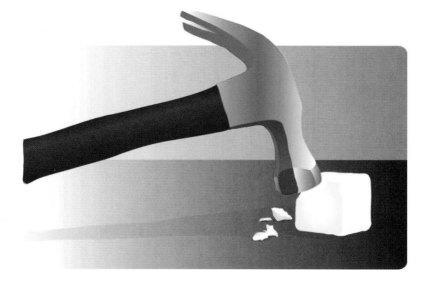

DEATH BY SUGAR

Now you know how your body metabolizes SUGAR, and you also know that the liver will turn unused SUGAR into **FAT** to be stored in your **FAT** cells. What if you don't make changes? What are you likely to expect?

Overweight adults and children should be especially worried about their SUGAR intake. As we grow older, our metabolism slows, and the damage done by overeating SUGAR has taken a toll on our cells. Most overweight adults and many overweight children are already *insulin resistant* and are well on their way to type 2 diabetes.

Insulin resistance occurs when the cells simply say "no" to the insulin trying to open the door to the furnace. The pancreas senses the high glucose level in the blood, and it sends out another surge of insulin to deal with the problem. Too much insulin can constrict your arteries and put you at risk for heart attacks. Excess insulin also stimulates your brain to make you hungry, creating the vicious cycle of SUGAR cravings. Of course, all the excess SUGAR stimulates your liver to manufacture **FAT**. As you grow older, all of this leads to high blood pressure, high blood triglyceride levels, and low levels of good HDL cholesterol. Next step for you? Type 2 diabetes.

Type 2 diabetes occurs once the cells quit responding to the insulin from your pancreas. Congratulations—you are now a diabetic! You have literally eaten yourself into diabetes. Diabetes leads to all sorts of nasty consequences, including (but not limited to) heart attacks, strokes, deafness, blindness, kidney failure, limb amputations, and DEATH.

Do I have your attention yet?

The good news is that all of this can be reversible, or at least substantially improved, by maintaining a low-SUGAR lifestyle. Several studies have shown that people may be able to eat their way out of insulin resistance and type 2 diabetes. In a June 2006 article, "Low Carb Diet Has Lasting Benefits in Obese Type 2 Diabetics," published by *Medscape Today*, a 6-month study is reviewed in which 2 control groups, both overweight and both with type 2 diabetes, were observed. A control group ate a diet with substantially less SUGAR intake from carbohydrates than did the other group. Although the study was only 6 months long, the follow-up went on for 22 months. The conclusion of the study showed that after 1 year patients with type 2 diabetes eating a low-SUGAR diet all had a lower number of hypoglycemic episodes, reduced glycated hemoglobin levels, reduced triglyceride levels, and stable levels of total cholesterol.

These conclusions are direct result of a low carbohydrate diet and cannot be disputed. Cutting off SUGAR and foods that metabolize into SUGAR are a direct benefit on all fronts.

In another article, "Diabetes: America's Epidemic," written by Eileen M. Wright, M.D., Dr. Wright tells us that 2003 CDC statistics reveal that diabetes in the United States has increased by 61 percent since 1991! She reveals an estimated 17 million Americans are diabetic, producing an annual cost of almost $92 billion! Of course this doesn't include the immeasurable cost of our national loss of lives due directly to SUGAR.

I liked her approach to it all; she agrees with me that one must "cut the head off the snake" by restricting SUGAR intake from foods containing carbohydrates like SUGAR soda, starchy vegetables, breads, rice, grains, desserts, cookies, candy, cereals and pasta to name a few all of which can be labeled metabolic poisons for diabetics. In her article Dr. Wright advises successful treatment for all diabetics begins with maintaining normal blood SUGAR. Of course in order to maintain normal blood sugar one must restrict the intake of high-SUGAR foods.

This is the basic principle behind the **Fat to Skinny** program. Medications to restrict blood sugar will never take the place of maintaining a healthy blood sugar level through diet and exercise. She concludes her article by agreeing with me that type 2 diabetes is reversible with simple diet and lifestyle changes. If you'd like to read her article go to this web address: **www.gsmcweb.com/?p=36**.

As you can see, it's up to you

LIFE

or

DEATH by SUGAR.

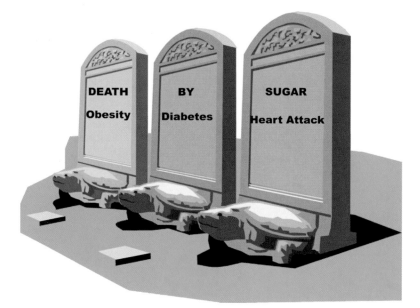

THE EXERCISE CONNECTION

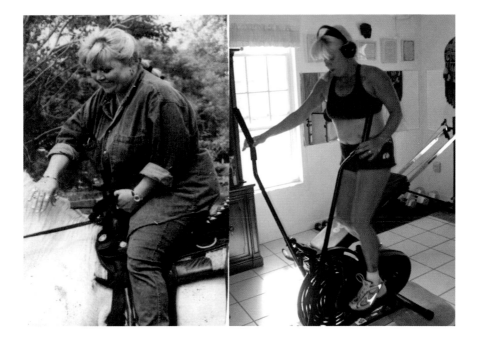

Don't exercise to lose weight! Eat **right** to lose weight. The above pictures are of my beautiful wife Sherri before a low-SUGAR eating plan, and then 70 pounds lighter after 6 months of low-SUGAR eating. She exercises for all the right reasons. She knows if you go into the gym or put on your jogging shoes to lose **FAT**, you're fighting an uphill battle. When you exercise to lose weight without changing your eating habits, you're simply battling your food intake.

Take, for example, our burger and medium order of fries. It takes 81 minutes of jogging at 5 mph to burn off the SUGAR derived from the hamburger bun and the fries! That's the wrong reason to be in the gym. You should exercise to build muscle, improve body tone, promote healthy circulatory and respiratory systems, increase your metabolism, and improve your attitude. Any weight loss you achieve from exercise is simply a bonus. Exercise does, however, increase the *speed* at which you'll lose **FAT** on this low-SUGAR program by increasing your metabolism. Your cells will require fuel from somewhere. Eating low-SUGAR forces the fuel to come from the stored **FAT**. Obviously, you would be far better off not eating the SUGAR to begin with. If you're eating the correct foods in balance with your everyday metabolism, you won't gain *any* **FAT** to burn off!

People who spend their lives working out to lose weight always end up **FAT** if they quit working out. Why? Because they don't change their eating habits. Here are some more examples of the amount of exercise required to simply burn off the SUGAR derived from the following foods:

25 minutes of aerobics for *each* pancake with syrup sitting in your pancake stack.

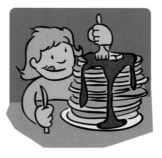

---

95 minutes of continuous swimming to burn off the SUGAR from an order of club sandwich and fries.

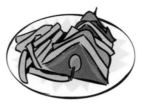

There is no SUGAR in the meat or the cheese, and there's very little in the veggies. The only SUGAR is coming from the bread and the fries.

190 minutes of golf to burn off a personal pan pizza. There is no SUGAR in the cheese or the meat toppings. All of the SUGAR is coming from the pizza crust (and a few from the veggies and sauce).

It's all about choices. If you schedule your banana or your apple or your slice of pizza to coincide with an activity suited to burn off *all* the SUGAR intake, then that SUGAR won't turn into **FAT**. Once you've lost all the **FAT** you want, scheduled exercise will be a wonderful way to allow you to increase your carbohydrate intake without gaining **FAT**. Be careful of the trap, however. Most people can't stick to an exercise regimen long term. If you rebuild your bad eating habits again by adding high-SUGAR foods back into your life and then quit working out, you'll get **FAT** again.

I don't worry about working out. I know that my everyday routine and my current SUGAR intake are in balance. For me, it's easier not to eat the bagel or the potato than it is to be forced into the gym by the food. *Always* eating low-SUGAR has allowed me the freedom to *choose* whether I want to work out on a particular day instead of being *forced* to work out by my SUGAR intake.

I know I'm a person who doesn't particularly like working out, and the gym comes in spurts for me. Usually, when I'm loaded with energy and stuck inside on a rainy day, my normal routine has me up and moving around. I'm doing something almost all the time. The only time I'm sedentary is in the evening or when I'm writing. You'll have to determine what kind of a person you are and whether exercise will play a part in your life. Some people are busy, but actually have less than physically active lifestyles; for example, the person who gets out of bed, drives to work, and sits, only to arrive back home by car to an easy chair. This is a person whose body has stayed fairly inactive all day long. This person needs to—at least—go for an evening stroll with the family pooch.

You need to be a realist. If you've failed up until now at keeping a scheduled exercise program in your life, then chances are you'll fail again. This is all the more reason NOT to put SUGAR into your body. I recommend exercise for all the right reasons, and fighting SUGAR intake in the gym isn't one of them. If you make the changes in your eating habits outlined in this book and eliminate SUGAR from your food intake, even the most sedentary person will lose **FAT**. If you're an active to very active person, you'll lose **FAT** faster. If you add some form of additional exercise into the mix, your weight loss will be even quicker. Simple arithmetic: The more fuel you burn, the faster the storage areas shrink. Exercise is *your* choice.

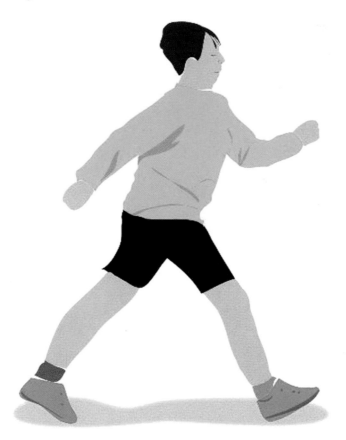

DON'T I NEED CARBOHYDRATES?

Yes, most definitely. Your brain and every one of your cells need carbohydrates to function properly. Modern science believes that the *average person* weighing in at a weight corresponding to their size and gender *and* maintaining a *"normal"* activity level needs upwards of 130 carbohydrates a day for proper cell and brain function. Is that you?

Everyone is different. Numbers like those are based on averages. I certainly could not eat that level of SUGAR on a daily basis and maintain my current 32-inch waist! As mentioned earlier, my SUGAR intake needs to be kept at around 20 carbs per day. I am not sedentary; I live an active lifestyle, and you'll only occasionally see me in the gym. I consider myself of *normal* weight for my size: 165 pounds at 5'11". I also consider my activity level to be *normal*, so I don't fit into these guidelines. You probably don't, either, considering you're reading this book.

You'll have your chance to find out how much SUGAR you can eat once you've lost the **FAT**. Believe me, right now you have plenty of carbohydrates stored around your body that need to be burned before you start to replace them by mouth. Once you have become SKINNY by burning the **FAT** stores in your body, it will be important to start replacing your carbohydrates by mouth. The difference is you'll be giving your body the *best* carbohydrates by eating complex carbs found in whole grains and vegetables, plus simple carbs found in fruit, all of it in measured and controlled quantities. You'll know when you reach your personal metabolic threshold for SUGAR intake by keeping an eye on the scale. If your normal daily routine doesn't burn all the SUGAR you take in, you'll start to gain weight again. When that happens, you'll know you're above your threshold and you'll need to cut back until your body starts to lose weight again. Use your scale once a week in the morning, and keep track of your progress with a log.

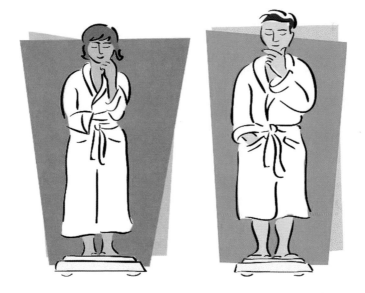

Make sure you keep a log and weigh yourself on a scheduled basis at the same time each week. This is especially important when you've lost all the weight you want. Ten pounds can come on quickly if you jump back into the SUGAR pipeline! The scale will keep you on your game.

SUGAR, THE GREAT BIG **FAT** LIE!

SUGAR is BIG business and does more than make us **FAT** around the midsection. SUGAR is responsible for many industries having **FAT** bottom lines! Christopher Columbus first introduced SUGAR to the new world at the end of the 14th century. By the 17th century, SUGAR production in the subtropical and tropical regions of the Americas had become the largest and most lucrative industry in the world. According to the U.S. Department of Commerce reports, SUGAR fuels (to name a few)…

Candy industry ($43 BILLION annual sales)

Soda pop industry ($70 BILLION in annual sales)

Snack industry ($57 BILLION in annual sales)

Diet industry ($35 BILLION in annual sales)

The International Sugar Journal reports, the U.S. SUGAR industry is one of the largest in the world generating over 146,000 jobs. This industry is responsible for almost $10 BILLION in economic activity in the 19 states where sugar beets and sugarcane is grown and processed.

Now let's take a look at the economic impact of **type 2 diabetes**. According to the National Library of Medicine, costs to the nation are now approaching $20 billion. Not to mention the terrible toll it takes on the afflicted. And this is just the tip of the iceberg when it comes to how SUGAR-related diseases affect the medical industry. UNTOLD BILLIONS are spent annually by our population on afflictions which ultimately can be traced back to our insatiable addiction to SUGAR.

The facts seem undeniable: *economically*, our country is far better off if we are **FAT** and obese than it is if we are thin and slender. Our nation's SUGAR addiction fuels way too much business. I'm afraid you won't get any help from the government on this problem anytime soon, either; all you have to do is review the following **NEW** food pyramid proposed by the US government. I went to the government's food pyramid website. They have a page where I could enter my statistics and they would send me MY pyramid.

www.mypyramid.gov/mypyramid/index.aspx

The website then calculated a "custom food pyramid" for me. It's LOADED with SUGAR! If I were to eat a diet relying on this information, I would be **FAT** as a cow in very short order and my SUGAR addiction would continue to be fueled. As you review my food pyramid, you'll notice the plan calls for me to consume the following foods on a weekly basis:

7 cups of grain	sugar
12 cups of high-carb veggies	sugar
14 cups of fruit	sugar

21 cups of low-fat milk	sugar
3 cups of beans, peas, nuts & seeds	sugar
3 cups of meat, fish or poultry	PROTEIN

It makes me wonder why the obvious and simplistic nutritional changes to lean out our nation are being completely ignored. Could it be economically driven? I'll leave that up to you to decide.

Doug's Custom Food Pyramid

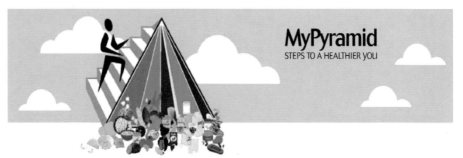

Based on the information you provided, this is your daily recommended amount from each food group.

GRAINS 8 ounces	VEGETABLES 3 cups	FRUITS 2 cups	MILK 3 cups	MEAT & BEANS 6 1/2 ounces
Make half your grains whole	**Vary your veggies**	**Focus on fruits**	**Get your calcium-rich foods**	**Go lean with protein**
Aim for at least **4 ounces** of whole grains a day	Aim for these amounts each week:	Eat a variety of fruit	Go low-fat or fat-free when you choose milk, yogurt, or cheese	Choose low-fat or lean meats and poultry
	Dark green veggies = 3 cups	Go easy on fruit juices		Vary your protein routine— choose more fish, beans, peas, nuts, and seeds
	Orange veggies = 2 cups			
	Dry beans & peas = 3 cups			
	Starchy veggies = 6 cups			
	Other veggies = 7 cups			

Find your balance between food and physical activity

Be physically active for at least **30 minutes** most days of the week.

Know your limits on fats, sugars, and sodium

Your allowance for oils is **7 teaspoons a day.**

Limit extras–solid fats and sugars–to **360 calories a day.**

Your results are based on a 2400 calorie pattern.   Name: _____

This calorie level is only an estimate of your needs. Monitor your body weight to see if you need to adjust your calorie intake.

Now let's compare my food pyramid to the diet of a meat steer. Is it possible people are eating COW FOOD? Author and small-scale cattleman Michael Pollan recently wrote about steer No. 534 in *The New York Times*. He followed No. 534 from birth to the slaughterhouse. In his article, entitled "Power Steer," he states that he fed No. 534 a daily diet of "14 pounds of corn and 6 pounds of hay—and added 2½ pounds every day to No. 534…On Nov. 13 he weighed 650 pounds; by Christmas he was up to 798…No. 534 put away 706 pounds of corn and 336 pounds of alfalfa hay." It's no secret that cow food is front-loaded with grains and corn to fatten up the cow for slaughter. After all, the rancher and everyone else get paid by the pound! GRAINS = SUGAR, SUGAR then turns into **FAT**. As I mentioned earlier, if I ate the diet plan outlined for me in my custom food pyramid, I would be as **FAT** as a COW! WHY? Because I would be eating COW FOOD. Cows eat corn and grains. Flour comes from ground GRAIN.

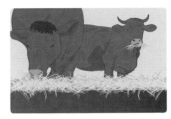 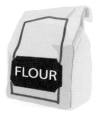

Flour is then processed into a zillion things, including bread, cookies, cake, bagels, tortillas, pasta, snacks, pretzels etc., etc., etc. It's ALL cow food!

Ever notice how sleek and streamlined the great cats are? Panthers, leopards, lions, and tigers. They don't eat COW food. They are carnivores, and they eat protein. We are carnivores as well. You'll lean out quickly if you switch from COW food to protein.

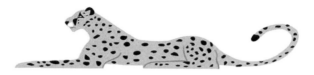

The key to ALL this **FAT** loss is a lifelong...
CHANGE OF EATING HABITS.

But are you really ready for that change? Addiction is addiction, whether you're talking about drugs, alcohol, or SUGAR. It all begins in your mind. Like sex, chocolate, and many drugs, SUGAR is believed by researchers to cause the brain to release dopamine in the pleasure centers of the brain, which then fuels the addiction.

According to the National Library of Medicine, daily bingeing on SUGAR repeatedly releases dopamine in the accumbens shell.

Simply spoken, SUGAR releases the "feel-good hormone" into your brain, fueling your desires for more SUGAR! It's a never-ending cycle. It's going to be completely up to you to re-train yourself to eat the foods that won't fuel your addiction and that won't make you **FAT**.

Your current eating habits are loaded with SUGAR. This is why the addiction has occurred in the first place, and this is why, at least up until now, being **FAT** has not been your fault. Now the question is, what are you going to do about it? Are you going to ignore the addiction like millions of others, or are you going to take action? Are you going to control your food intake with good choices? It's really easier than you might think. Most of the time, eating low-SUGAR is not about what you put *on* a plate as much as what you take *off* a plate. Use this book and labels to learn how to identify the SUGAR in the ingredients and it will be easy for you to make those choices.

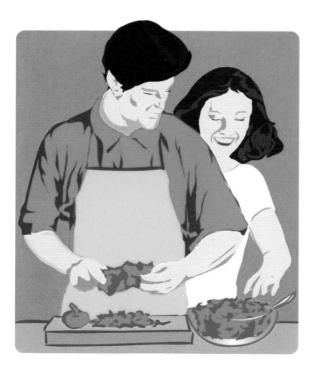

THE PSYCHOLOGICAL CONNECTION

Change is scary, even when it's for our own good. People like their *groove*; it fits like an old shoe. You not only have the issue of recognizing your SUGAR addiction to deal with, but you also have the other members of your household—who also have some level of SUGAR addiction—to deal with. They want to eat what *they* want to eat, not what you tell them to eat. Your problem is not their problem. To make matters worse, you'll have to take TOTAL charge of the foods that go into your mouth at home, at work, at dinner parties, and at restaurants. You'll need to be disciplined enough to stick to the good foods and have the strength to avoid the ones that have—and will continue to make you—**FAT**. Those foods will ALWAYS be at your fingertips wherever you go. In short, for you to succeed in your quest to become SKINNY, it needs to be important enough to you to make the appropriate changes in your eating habits.

Will it be difficult? All change comes with some level of difficulty; it depends on *your* personal commitment. For those of you who are determined to do something about your **FAT** problem once and for all, it will be easy, and you'll never be hungry. You simply have to make the changes required in your ingredient intake. Think of your personal battle with weight loss over the years. Us **FAT** people are willing to do just about anything to lose weight, except give up the foods we think we love.

I say "think" we love because you'll be amazed at how lousy white mashed potatoes, pasta, and white bread *really* taste once you remove them from your daily intake. But *wanting* to get SKINNY and *doing something* about getting SKINNY are totally separate issues. Millions of people *want* to be zillionaires, as long as it's a lottery win and they don't have to work for it. Millions of alcoholics *want* to quit drinking, but not bad enough to throw away the bottle. The amazing thing about getting rid of SUGAR is how simple the process is. The difficult part for most SUGAR addicts is actually doing it. Many people would rather do some of the things I have listed below. You may have tried one or several of the following methods yourself:

LOW-FAT DIETS

STARVING YOURSELF

TAKING DIET PILLS

AN ALL-LIQUID DIET

CONSIDERING LIPOSUCTION

KILLING YOURSELF IN THE GYM

CONSIDERING GASTRIC BYPASS

or worse

GIVING UP COMPLETELY!

In light of the above, spending a little time and effort on what you're actually eating that's *causing* your **FAT** problem doesn't seem so bad, now, does it? Think about it this way: If you were allergic to peanuts, and eating even the smallest amount could kill you, would you eat them? Of course not! And SUGAR *is* killing you as sure as peanuts kill some people. The only difference is that it's killing you *slowly*.

Eliminating SUGAR from your system will never be easier or better for you. You'll become thin and energetic, and you'll look and feel better, all without being hungry. You'll be able to dine out at most restaurants by giving instructions to the waitstaff. You'll be able to carry foods with you that will satisfy your body's needs without causing you to become **FAT**. You'll be able to enjoy many of your favorite recipes with some substitutions. This is your moment of truth. Moving forward from here can and will be your miracle, if you're ready for it.

What is your motivation to lose weight? Funny enough, mine was that one day I would no longer be a *special person*. I simply wanted to be a *normal person*, a person who could walk the beach in a Speedo bathing suit and not look ridiculous. Little did I know growing up that, as an adult, reaching the Speedo wish I had struggled with since I was 8 or 9 years old would be my motivator.

I have spoken to lots of people about motivation. Some are motivated because they want to live to play with their grandchildren. Some are motivated strictly by vanity or health. Others are motivated because they had given up and now see the possibility of finally getting SKINNY. Whatever your motivation, write it down on a Post-it note and stick it on your fridge. Find your goal-orientated self and charge forward.

My **FAT** friends thought I was crazy when I started eating low-SUGAR. I got all the negative comments. "Your heart's going to blow eating all that food!" "You're crazy! You can't eat all that food and lose weight!" Believe me, I enjoyed myself thoroughly as 50 pounds melted away like butter in a hot pan in just 4 months. My **FAT** melted so fast I actually had a friend ask me if I had contracted AIDS! I laughed, and we sat and talked about eating low-SUGAR/low-carb. The guy who was calling me crazy just a short 4 months earlier was now VERY curious about how I had lost all that **FAT**! He now wanted the secrets to losing his *ORB*. That's what he called his gut, his ORB. And his ORB was growing bigger every day. Five months later, he was 40 pounds lighter without exercise and while eating all the food he wanted. My friend dropped down to 175 pounds and ate ice cream all the way down! *Did I say ice cream?*

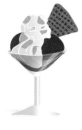

There is one more chemical issue to discuss with you. Remember what I said: You need to keep your **net** carbohydrate intake to under 20 grams per day to shed the **FAT**. There is a difference between carbohydrates and **net** carbohydrates. It's the word **NET** that we need to discuss. Some carbohydrates don't cause an insulin spike. Those carbs are SUGAR alcohols, artificial sweeteners, and fiber. When determining your carb counts in foods, you need to subtract SUGAR alcohols and fiber from the total carb count on labels to arrive at **net** carbs. This is important to you because it opens up many foods to you that otherwise would be avoided, including candy. Yes, I said candy. ALWAYS check the labels of everything you eat until the statistics are like second nature to you. Here's an example of a typical label and how you'll arrive at your net carb count:

NUTRITION FACTS
Serving size 1 bar (30 grams)

Calories	120
Calories from Fat	45
Total Fat	5g
Saturated Fat	3g
Trans fat	0g
Cholesterol	<5mg
Sodium	70mg
Total Carbohydrates	**15g**
Dietary Fiber	2g
Sugars	<1g
Sugar Alcohol	12g
Protein	6g

Total Carbohydrates   1 gram

This is a Slim Fast snack bar sweetened with the SUGAR alcohol Splenda. In this example, one bar is the serving size. Total carbs listed is 15 grams. Subtract 2 grams of fiber and 12 grams of SUGAR alcohol for a final net carb count of **1**. You could eat this bar and still have 19 grams of net carbs to play with for the day.

See how easy that was? **READ LABELS!** Here is a SUGAR-free Jell-O label—no carbs, no SUGAR!

NUTRITION FACTS
Serving size ¼ package (2.5 grams)

Calories	10
Total Fat	0g
Saturated Fat	0g
Trans Fat	0g
Sodium	55mg
Total Carbohydrates	**0g**
Sugars	0g
Protein	1g

Total Carbohydrates   0 grams

LET'S DISCUSS SUGAR ALCOHOLS AND ARTIFICIAL SWEETENERS

OK, so you have a sweet tooth and find yourself in need of an occasional fix, what do you do? Obviously SUGAR is out of the question . . . but good news is on the horizon. You can have your sweets and still lose weight.

SUGAR alcohols and artificial sweeteners are what sweeten SUGAR-free products, including SUGAR-free candy, ice cream, and soda. They come in several forms, including stevia, malitol, acesulfame potassium, sucralose (Splenda), sorbitol, saccharin, aspartame (Nutrasweet), mannitol, xylitol, lactitol, and isomalt.

There are a few things you should know about SUGAR alcohols and artificial sweeteners. First of all, they are reported not to have any significant effect on blood SUGAR. Some will, however, burn as fuel before **FAT** does. There are conflicting reports regarding their effects on different people. For example, some diabetics report a SUGAR *high* from some of these products, and some diabetic doctors require their patients to be wary of their use. I have been successful using these products as long as I keep them to a minimum. SUGAR-free products are your rewards and should be eaten as **occasional treats**, and not on a daily basis. It's also important to stay within the serving size. Most diet soda is sweetened with aspartame or Splenda. I prefer the Splenda-sweetened soda to the aspartame-sweetened soda. I've identified aspartame in my diet as a major cause of headaches, so I keep its use to a minimum.

Aspartame is by far the most controversial of all artificial sweeteners so I'm going to spend a little extra time discussing it with you. Stories abound on the web about its ill effects. As you read their stories, the authors will try to convince you that this artificial sweetener is as bad as ingesting radioactive material. I'm not a scientist so I can only comment truthfully to you about my personal experience with the stuff. If you're experiencing headaches and using the little blue packets or drinking diet soda sweetened with aspartame, try eliminating them from your diet. You may be surprised when your headaches suddenly disappear.

Of course I wouldn't be satisfied advising you without some fairly exhaustive research on the subject. I went straight to the top and bypassed the doomsday articles written by *people*, many of whom are unqualified to write them in the first place. Instead I read study after study performed by scientists, clinical labs and medical professionals. What conclusion did I come to? The FDA, the manufacturer, and many clinical studies claim that aspartame is perfectly safe, while many reports, watchdog groups, and web sites claim we are all being poisoned for the sake of corporate profits.

Who do you believe, the guys making money from the sales of product or the watchdog groups trying to save the world?

You decide. Below I've supplied you with the web addresses for the manufacturer of aspartame, the FDA report on artificial sweeteners including aspartame, and the web addresses for a couple of sites claiming aspartame is bad for you. I've also included the study performed by the National Cancer Institute. This will allow you to determine your personal position on aspartame. *My position* is simple: the stuff causes me headaches so I don't use it. There are simply too many other products available sweetened with far less controversial sweeteners to choose from, so why take the chance.

Sites for Aspartame Safety

http://www.aboutaspartame.com/professional/index.asp

http://www.fda.gov/FDAC/features/1999/699_sugar.html

Sites Condemning Aspartame

http://www.medicalnewstoday.com/articles/34040.php

http://www.holisticmed.com/aspartame/

National Cancer Institute Study

http://www.cancer.gov/cancertopics/factsheet/risk/aspartame

Malitol and sorbitol are major sweeteners in SUGAR-free candies, carb-free protein bars, and carb-free ice cream. The major side effect from these sweeteners is flatulence. Too much of a good thing will cause you to have gas (or worse), so take it easy and stay within the suggested serving size.

Stevia is my chosen sweetener; it's all natural, it has no carbs in its pure form and therefore doesn't need to be counted. Stevia can be purchased at most health food stores in several forms. Be careful to check the labels on the form you choose. I have found stevia in packets that have additional ingredients added to create more of a granular effect. It's the additional ingredients that can bring carbs into the product. In its raw form, it's more like baby powder. I sweeten my coffee, so I prefer the stevia tablets. I buy them on the web at **www.sweetleaf.com**. They also sell the other forms of the product.

I recommend you limit your SUGAR-free sodas to no more than 4 per day, spread out through the day. Make water your main source of hydration. What I do is open a can of soda and top off my water glass with a splash of soda. One can of soda goes a long way using this method. You can eat a measured serving of Breyers CarbSmart ice cream or SUGAR-free candy no more than 3 times per week. I enjoy a serving of SUGAR-free Jell-O topped with Reddi-wip more than any of the other desserts. This dessert can be eaten every day.

If your weight loss plateaus for longer than 2 weeks, eliminate ALL SUGAR alcohol and artificially sweetened products from your intake. Once you start dropping weight again, slowly add back the *necessity* products and keep an eye on the scale. You may discover some sweeteners affect your weight and others don't.

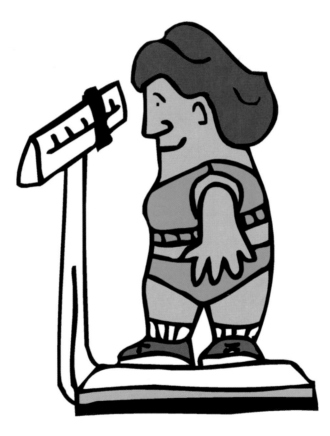

EATING YOURSELF SKINNY

By now you're probably asking yourself what you'll be able to eat that will be good for you and not feed into your SUGAR addiction. Let's start with 2 rules:

Eat MEATS and GREENS to grow THIN and LEAN

Eat SUGAR and CARBS to grow FAT and LARGE

Coming up in the next chapter of this book is your new ingredient list for your household shopping. Before you go to the store, I want you to analyze ALL of the food in your house. Read EVERY label on every bit of food you have in your cabinets and refrigerator. It's time to clean house of all the stuff that's making you **FAT**. Box up EVERYTHING that has a net carb count of over 4 grams per serving. Remember, net carbs are arrived at by looking at the total carb count on the label and subtracting the fiber and the SUGAR alcohols. The SUGAR that's listed on the label is factored into the total carb count and is *not subtracted*. ***Only the fiber and the SUGAR alcohols get subtracted from the total carb count to arrive at net carbs.***

Next, return what you can to your grocery store and give the non-returnable, sealed items to charity. Throw the rest away! If you're going to shut off the SUGAR pipeline, it begins at home. Everyone in your home will benefit from this eating plan—even the thin people living with you. You can save those thin people from becoming **FAT**, unless of course you want them to experience being a *special person* at Joubert's. ☺

Next, take this book to the store and restock your house with ALL low-SUGAR foods. It's time to eat yourself SKINNY! Some products will not be available at your grocery store and will need to be ordered in by phone or over the web. Get used to it; as the low-carb FAD dies away, so will the low-carb products being carried in your local store. For us, shopping on the web has become part of the norm. To make it easier for you, I have provided you with the ordering information. A word of caution: *carefully read labels*. Something advertised as "SUGAR-free" may still be loaded with hidden SUGAR. The only measurement that's important to you is the NET CARBOHYDRATE COUNT.

SAMPLE LABEL

Total Carbohydrates	24g
Dietary Fiber	6g
Sugar	5g
Sugar Alcohols	10g

NET CARBS   8g

Carbs (24) - [Fiber (6) + SUGAR Alcohols (10)] = 8

WHEN SHOULD YOU EAT?

When you eat and how much you eat is determined by your activity level and your portion control. Whoever came up with the ritual of breakfast, lunch, and dinner based on the clock was an idiot. Your body requires energy to burn when you're burning energy. It doesn't require high doses of food if you're sedentary, any more than your car requires more gas when it's not running. Take the BEAR, for example. During hibernation, the bear slows down its metabolism and lives on body **FAT**. Are you hibernating or are you running all day long? Active people will need to eat more frequently than non-active people.

Before we discuss suggested eating times and quantities, let's discuss hunger. Do you know what the feeling of hunger is? Are you eating because it's your lunch break, or are you eating because you're hungry? Does your body tell you you're hungry and *then* you think of food, or do you think of food and *then* become hungry? For example, have you ever walked past a bakery and smelled *that bakery smell* and THEN said, "That smells wonderful. I'm hungry"? That's an example of food giving you false hunger. An example of true hunger is when your body interrupts you with signals and actually *tells you it's hungry. Note: a growling stomach may be a false signal of hunger brought on by years of scheduled feedings.* The best way to determine when you're truly hungry is to experience hunger in your own body and learn from the signals. For some people, stomach growls are enough. Others experience a feeling of low energy, others get cold, and others get grumpy.

The best thing to do is start off with a 3-day test. (Yes, you need a paper and pencil.) Start your morning off with a small breakfast of 2 eggs, 3 strips of bacon or ham, and 2 pieces of GG Bran CrispBread with 2 tablespoons of the peanut butter mixture from the ingredient section. For a beverage, drink whatever you want as long as it's SUGAR-free. Now write down the time you ate. Next, head into your day and see what happens. When you start to feel hunger, analyze it. Is it hunger or habit? Did you start thinking of food and that's what made you feel hungry, or were you interrupted by your body *telling you* you're hungry?

If your body has interrupted you from your work and told you you're hungry, then listen to it. If you started thinking about food and *then* became hungry, then you're experiencing a craving. Either way, write down the time on your paper and note whether it's true hunger or a craving. If it's a craving, drink a large glass of water or 2 and the craving will pass. If it's hunger, it will come back fairly quickly. If it's true hunger, have a small snack from any of the items on your ingredient list. It doesn't matter whether it's a handful of almonds, a couple of pieces of beef jerky, a hard-boiled egg, or items from the veggie tray. Now wait 15 to 20 minutes for the body to register the food and see how you feel. If you're satisfied the hunger has passed, make a note of what time you ate, what you ate, and the quantity of what you ate. If you're still hungry after 20 minutes, eat a little bit more and wait another 15 minutes, making notes along the way.

Once you've satisfied your hunger, it's time to wait for the body to signal you again. You may not hear from your body for another 4 or 5 hours, or you may hear from your body within 2 hours. It all depends on your activity level. Ignore the breakfast, lunch, and dinner schedule for 3 full days.

The only scheduled meal I want you to eat during this experiment is breakfast, and I don't want you to eat *that* until you're hungry! It may be 10 a.m. before your body is asking for food. If you get an early start in the morning and usually don't eat breakfast until 10 a.m., that's OK. Hard-boiled eggs are the same as fried eggs, and you can carry them with you. Eat when you get your first *true* hunger. That will start your day with a timeline to work from. If you reach lunchtime and find you're not truly hungry, don't eat! Wait for the signals. It may be 2 in the afternoon before you feel hunger. That's when you'll eat another snack, and then wait for the signals again. Again, keep a log of your body's commands and responses.

After continuing with this experiment for 3 full days, you'll know when your feeding times are based on your log and the responses your body had to the food. Your goal during this 3-day experiment is to put yourself in direct contact with your body's true feeding times verses cravings, and to identify the true quantity of food your body requires to satisfy those needs.

Once you have finished your experiment, look at the feeding schedule you experienced over 3 days. You should discover that you get urges to eat at about the same time each day. You'll also discover that it doesn't take much food to satisfy your needs during those times. Now you can custom schedule *your* feedings to *your* feeding times, and maybe even rejoin the lunch and dinner crowd. To rejoin the lunch and dinner crowd, analyze your snack times and see how they coincide with the scheduled lunch and dinner breaks. For example, if you ate your breakfast at 8:30 a.m. and didn't get hungry again until 11 a.m. during your 3-day experiment, you know that your body gets hungry an hour before the noon lunch break. You'll deal with this by eating a small amount at 11 a.m. Now, when lunchtime rolls around, you won't feel ravenous and you'll eat a smaller feeding at lunchtime. Three hours later your next feeding time may come up from your log. That's OK—have a small snack from the list to tide you over until dinner, and then eat a smaller dinner.

For Sherri and me, our eating schedule is as follows:

GG Bran CrispBread & peanut butter with coffee, 7 a.m.
Breakfast or brunch—between 10 a.m. and 11 a.m.

Snacks—between 2 p.m. and 3 p.m.
Dinner—between 5 p.m. and 6 p.m.
Ice cream or Jell-O—8 p.m.

We eat 5 smaller meals per day instead of 3 big meals. Each of you will be different based on your experiment. Once you know your personal hunger schedule, you'll be prepared for it and will have food ready to eat on time. This will stop the ravenous search for something to eat when you're over-hungry and couldn't care less what goes into your mouth.

Don't let anyone make you feel that you're doing something wrong if you don't sit down at the food trough on someone else's schedule. This is *your* body, *your* schedule. There's nothing antisocial about it. You do what's right for you, not what's right for someone else. Just because dinner is on the table doesn't mean that you have to join in the feed. If you're not truly hungry, don't eat! Once you begin this practice you'll get to know your timelines so well that you'll never be hungry again. You'll eat when you first sense the feelings, satisfying your needs. And you'll never be ravenous.

During your experiment, you may also discover other reasons that you're eating. It's important to recognize the signs, because you may be *emotionally* eating. Pain seeks pleasure, and for SUGAR addicts, food *is* pleasure. If you find yourself seeking food because you're mad or upset, sad or stressed-out, then you're seeking pleasure from food to reverse the pain from the event. You are *emotionally* eating. This is simply a habit, and all habits can be broken if you recognize them. The trick is to replace the bad habit with a good habit. Find something besides food to bring you pleasure in times like these. Learn to eat for the right reasons. My personal demon is *nervous* eating. I call it "mindless" eating because I'm doing it without realizing it. If I have anxiety about something, I find myself strolling around the kitchen (and inevitably, to the fridge). For me, it's imperative to "bullet-proof" my kitchen and my fridge with SUGAR-free snacks.

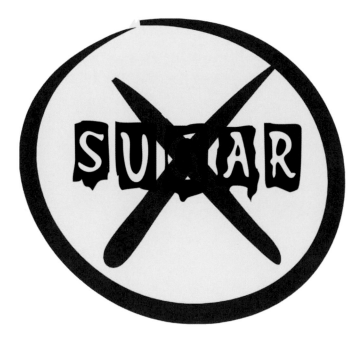

I'M STARVING!
TIME FOR A SNACK.

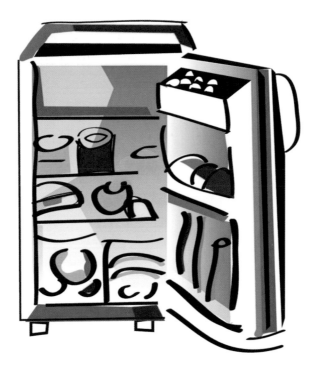

You've read a lot, I've written a lot. Let's share a snack together. I'll show you how easy it can be. Take me to your fridge!

Eating low-SUGAR is all about choices. Look for lunch meats like ham or sliced turkey. Grab the sliced cheese and the jar of pickles. Put all that stuff on the counter. Now lay out a piece of sandwich meat on a plate. On top of that, put a piece of cheese. Now lay a ¼ pickle slice on top of the cheese and roll the whole thing up like a sleeping bag. Congratulations, you're a chef! You just made a "meat, pickle, and cheese rollup." The only place SUGAR can be is if the meat is glazed with SUGAR or if there's SUGAR in the pickles. Check the labels. Buy SUGAR-free dill pickles, and deli meats without any SUGAR or honey glaze. Mix and match and include olives, if you wish. Keep rollups in the fridge ALL the time so you have something to grab when you're hungry.

Are you ready for another one?

Take out the eggs and hard-boil them. Once they're cooled and peeled, you can enjoy them whole with salt and pepper. Or you can make deviled eggs by cutting them in half lengthwise, taking out the yolk, mixing the yolks with some mayo (check the label), and stuffing the mixture back into the egg white. BINGO, deviled eggs! Keep these at your fingertips, too.

Got any hot dogs? Grab one and pop it in a microwave-safe bowl with a little water in the bottom. Cover with plastic wrap and microwave for a couple of minutes.

Take out a head of lettuce and peel off a big leaf. Put in some mustard, put in your hot dog, roll it up, and eat it. Your catsup is probably full of SUGAR, so check the label. If you like catsup, buy SUGAR-free catsup. It's available at most stores.

While the lettuce and the lunchmeat and the boiled eggs are still out, let's make a nice big chef's salad for lunch. Put a mess of greens into a bowl, top it off with slivers of meats and cheeses and a hard-boiled egg. Check the dressings in the fridge. A lot of your favorites already in there are probably low-carb.

Do you have any shrimp in the freezer? Boil some up in Old Bay seasoning and leave them in the fridge to snack on. Mix some of that SUGAR-free catsup with some horseradish to make a SUGAR-free cocktail sauce. Let's check the veggie drawer. Pull out the broccoli, celery, cucumber, radishes, yellow squash, and the zucchini. Cut up a nice mix of this stuff and make yourself a low-SUGAR veggie tray. Use the low-SUGAR dressings in the fridge as a dip.

Let's check the freezer. See any boneless chicken breasts? Take a couple out and pan-fry them in some olive oil. Once cooled, slice them up, put some salt and pepper on them, and keep them in a bowl in the fridge. While we're in the freezer, let's check on steak. If you see a steak in the freezer, slice it up and then stick the meat strips on bamboo skewers. These are great grilled and left in the fridge. We love "meat on a stick!" If, by chance, you have any Walden Farms SUGAR-free BBQ sauce in the cabinet, brush some on during grilling.

We have lots of stuff out on the counter, so let's make one more thing together. Let's make kabobs! All you have to do is put chunks of chicken or steak on the bamboo skewers along with chunks of yellow and green squash, a piece of onion, a couple of pieces of bell pepper, and on the grill they go.

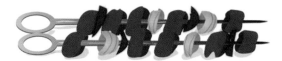

See how easy that was? Your fridge is now LOADED with healthy SUGAR-free and low-SUGAR treats. Get into the habit of making your own snack trays every day so you always have picking food. A mixture of these items can end up in your fridge at the office very easily.

When planning meals, plan on a main ingredient that can be used in different dishes for a couple of days. For example, let's say you plan a baked ham for Sunday dinner. Monday could be ham and eggs for breakfast, and *chicken cordon bleu* for dinner. *Chicken cordon bleu* is a chicken breast stuffed with ham and Swiss cheese, then baked. You'll find the recipe in the recipe section of this book. While you're making your *chicken cordon bleu*, prepare 2 or 3 extras. That way, you can slice them into pinwheels the next day and put them on a snack tray. Preparing food will become a habit for you. If you don't like to cook and prefer eating out, I have prepared a chapter further on in the book just for you.

INGREDIENT LIST

If you encounter problems with any product web addresses, refer to our website for updates.

DINNERS and LUNCHES

Fresh MEATS, POULTRY, FISH

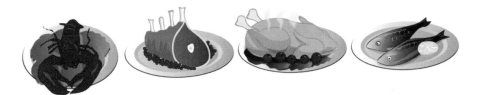

Buy any kind of meat, poultry, or fish you want, as long as it's lean, fresh, and not processed with store marinades or coatings. They are all *0 net carbs*. **Try to keep your serving size to 6 oz, but if you're still hungry after 15 minutes, EAT MORE.**

Carb-free doesn't mean calorie-free, and although this eating plan does not require you to count calories, portion sizes should be controlled to avoid gluttony. It takes the body longer to recognize the "full" feeling from protein, so try to eat a little slower and use the "15-minute rule" before refilling your plate with second helpings. Most people will feel full within 15 minutes with a 6 oz portion of protein.

Think of it. Steaks, chops, turkey, chicken, pork, roasts, salmon, grouper, shrimp, crab, tuna, crawfish, veal, lamb, and all the other wonderful non-processed fresh meats, poultry, and fish products contain ZERO SUGAR! Your dinner plate is starting off well, don't you think? Side the meat, poultry, or fish with a nice salad and any of the vegetables on the upcoming list for a complete, well-balanced, virtually SUGAR-free meal! Make wonderful chef's salads for lunches with GG Bran CrispBread as a side. Finish with a dessert of fresh strawberries, blackberries, or raspberries topped with Reddi-wip topping! Or, if you prefer, a ½ cup portion of Bryers CarbSmart ice cream or SUGAR-free Jell-O with Reddi-wip topping!

BREAKFASTS

BACON, SAUSAGE, and HAM

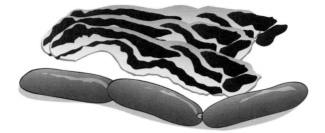

Most bacon, sausage, and ham are zero (or very low) in net carbs. **Check the labels** and beware of *SUGAR-cured* or *SUGAR-coated* products; they are loaded with carbs. I also still practice eating foods with the lowest possible **FAT** content to maintain healthy cholesterol levels. Buy leaner cuts and lower **FAT** content products as long as there is no added SUGAR. Enjoy bacon and eggs for breakfast as often as you wish. Help control cholesterol by substituting whole eggs with Egg Beaters, and replace pork bacon with Louis Rich Turkey Bacon. Replace the toast with GG Bran CrispBread. Enjoy cheese omelets and soufflés. On the run, make BLTs and breakfast wraps made in La Tortilla Factory tortillas or wrapped in romaine leaves.

EGGS, EGG BEATERS, and CHEESES

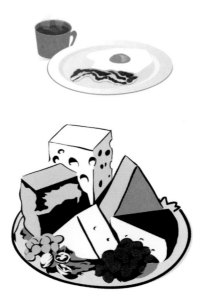

Buy any kind you want—they are all very low or *0 net carbs*, except for some **FAT**-free cheeses. Check the labels, and if they are under 2 net carbs per serving, they're OK. Discover the world of fine cheeses. You'll be amazed at the variety and selection of cheeses from around the world to explore, all of them SUGAR-free and loaded with calcium. To control cholesterol, limit whole eggs by using egg substitutes, such as Egg Beaters, and watch your portion sizes with full-**FAT** cheeses. Info on Egg Beaters can be found at **www.eggbeaters.com**.

BEVERAGES

WATER *0 net carbs*

Diet soda *0 net carbs, limit to 4 per day*

Stick with brands of diet soda sweetened with Splenda or Stevia; stay away from aspartame. Diet Rite made by RC Cola has 4 flavors: cola, white grape, black cherry, and orange. Coke and Pepsi also have certain sodas with Splenda.

Herbal teas   *0 net carbs*
Black coffee   *1 net carb*
Wyler's Light   *1 net carb*
Crystal Light   *1 net carb*

Lighten coffee with half & half (1 tbsp)   *.5 net carbs*
or heavy whipping cream   *0 net carbs*
Sweeten with stevia tabs   *0 net carbs*

BREADS

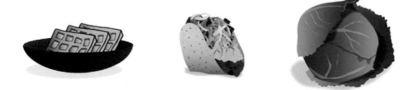

You'll need no other kind of bread besides GG Bran CrispBread and La Tortilla Factory tortillas, and nice crisp romaine lettuce leaves. There are several *crisp breads* on the market, many of them loaded with SUGAR, so I want you to buy the one I recommend. Order a case over the web and use it for peanut butter crackers, cheese and crackers, cream cheese and jelly, peanut butter and jelly (Frugeli brand jelly), or simply with butter or olive oil alongside a meal or salad. They are 100% bran, so they give you a good dose of fiber.

La Tortilla Factory tortillas are wonderful and come in 3 flavors. They are probably available from your local health food store or better grocery store, but if not, I've supplied the web address. They make terrific wraps for sandwiches. They also make great enchiladas and fajitas. We also use nice big fresh romaine lettuce leaves as a wrapper. We fill them with ham, turkey, salami and cheeses for fulfilling sandwiches that are totally carb-free. They also make for a great hamburger or hot dog bun replacement.

GG Bran CrispBread *2 net carbs*
www.brancrispbread.com

La Tortilla Factory Tortilla *3 net carbs*
www.latortillafactory.com

DESSERTS and JELLY

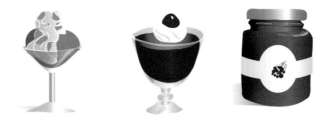

YES, desserts! Eat in moderation. I know you have a sweet tooth, so I've provided you with some prepackaged products sweetened with SUGAR alcohols or artificial sweeteners. Remember what I said about SUGAR alcohols: They are self-policing. Eat too many and they will cause a laxative affect. Stay within the portion size once or twice a day and you'll be fine.

Tastykake Sugar Free Sensables
Chocolate Chip Cake   *4 net carbs*
Chocolate Cake   *2 net carbs*
www.tastykake.com
Also available at Publix stores & Walmart.

Heavenly Desserts Sugar-free Meringue Cookies
Vanilla, chocolate, cappuccino, strawberry, and lemon, all *0 net carbs*
www.d-litefulbaking.com
Also available at Publix stores.

Frugeli Zero-sugar Jelly
Available in 3 flavors: grape, raspberry, and orange,
1 net carb per serving
www.sorbee.com

ICE CREAM, JELL-O, and WHIPPED CREAM

Available at most grocery stores

Breyers CarbSmart (½ cup) *4 net carbs*
Vanilla, butter pecan, chocolate, and rocky road.
You'll find these products on their web site under the
Breyers tab/packaged ice cream.
www.icecreamusa.com

Blue Bunny No Sugar Added (½ cup) *3 net carbs*
Peanut butter fudge, chocolate almond fudge. You'll find
these flavors on their web site under Lighter Options/No
Sugar Added, Reduced Fat Products.
www.bluebunny.com

Jell-O brand SUGAR-free gelatin *0 net carbs*
www.kraftfoods.com/jello/

Reddi-wip canned real whipped cream topping *<1 net carb*
www.reddi-wip.com

CANDY and COOKIES

Russell Stover SUGAR-free candy is wonderful. So are the **Hershey's** brand candies. Walmart stores carry both brands.
www.russellstover.com
www.hersheys.com

Heavenly Desserts Meringues *0 net carbs*
Strawberry, chocolate, vanilla, cappuccino, lemon
www.d-litefulbaking.com
Beanit Butter Walnut Cookies *0 net carbs*
Recipe in recipe section

FRUIT

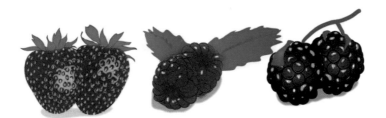

Fresh or frozen berries and avocados are the only fruits you're allowed until you've lost ALL the **FAT** you want. At that point, you can slowly add some of the other lower SUGAR fruits into your diet, such as apples, watermelon, cantaloupe, honeydew, apricots, and peaches. The following counts are for ½ cup servings unless otherwise noted:

Strawberries   **3.5 net carbs**
Blackberries   **5.5 net carbs**
Raspberries   **3 net carbs**
Avocado (small) **2 net carbs**

MUFFIN and PANCAKE MIXES

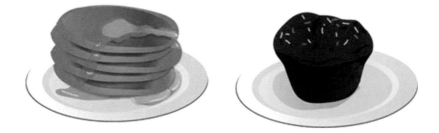

Top with cream cheese for a delicious treat.

Dixie Carb Counters
Banana nut muffin (1) **4 net carbs**
Carrot muffin mix (1) **1 net carb**
Cranberry orange muffin (1) **4 net carbs**
www.dixiediner.com

New Hope Mills Low Carb Sugar-Free Pancake & Waffle mix
(4 pancakes) **3 net carbs**
www.carbsmart.com

Log Cabin Sugar-Free Syrup
(¼ cup) **0 net carbs**
Available at most grocery stores

NUTS, CHIPS, and PEANUT BUTTER

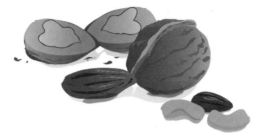

Dry Roasted Edamame (¼ cup) *2 net carbs*
www.seapointfarms.com

Almonds (30) *2.5 net carbs*

Walnuts (¼ cup) *1 net carb*

EatSmart Soy Crisps (10) *3 net carbs*
www.eatsmartsnacks.com

Pork Skins, fried, unsweetened *0 net carbs*

Peanut Butter, soy *0 net carbs*

Carb Not Beanit Butter *0 net carbs*
www.dixiediner.com
Order number (1-800-233-3668)

Smucker's Chunky Natural Peanut Butter
(2 tablespoons) *4 net carbs*

Doug's Crunchy Peanut Butter Mix—one 15 oz jar of Carb Not Beanit Butter mixed with one 16 oz jar of Smucker's Chunky Natural Peanut Butter and ½ cup chopped Dry Roasted Edamame (2 tbsp) *2 net carbs*

PROTEIN BARS

You have to be careful with protein bars. Many are loaded with SUGAR. I recommend the following:

Optimum Nutrition Complete Protein Diet Bars (1 bar)
1 net carb
www.optimumnutrition.com

SAUCES and SALAD DRESSING

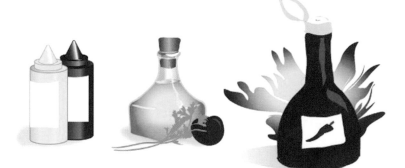

Walden Farms BBQ Sauces *0 net carbs*
www.waldenfarms.com

Bertolli Alfredo Sauce (¼ cup) *3 net carbs*

Winn-Dixie Pasta Sauce (¼ cup) *2 net carbs*

Emeril's Roasted Red Pepper Pasta Sauce (¼ cup) *2.5 net carbs*
www.everythingemeril.com

Heinz Classic Chicken Gravy (¼ cup) *3 net carbs*

Tabasco Hot Sauce *0 net carbs*

Cholula Hot Sauce *0 net carbs*

Bertolli Alfredo Sauce (¼ cup) *3 net carbs*
www.bertolli.com

Many brand-name salad dressings are already low in SUGAR. Check the labels on your favorites. Here are some examples:

Kraft Seven Seas (2 tbsp) **2 net carbs**

Kraft Classic Caesar (2 tbsp) *<1 net carbs*

Wish-Bone Carb-Options Blue Cheese (2 tbsp) *0 net carbs*

Athenos Greek with Feta Cheese (2 tbsp) *2 net carbs*

Sour cream (2 tbsp) *1 net carb*

PASTA

Tofu Shirataki Pasta (1 cup) *2 net carbs*
www.house-foods.com

VEGETABLES

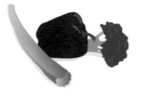

Look at the incredible amount of variety in your veggie list, all of it low in SUGAR! Get creative with your veggies. Make meat or seafood stir-fries, enjoy delectable chef's salads with eggs, cheeses, and meats. Enjoy steamed cauliflower run through your food processor as a mashed potato replacement. Enjoy spaghetti squash, julienned zucchini, or Tofu Shirataki Pasta as a replacement for pasta. Or simply enjoy veggie trays with ranch dressing as an anytime snack.

Counts are for ½ cup servings unless otherwise noted:

Artichoke hearts	*2 net carbs*
Asparagus, fresh (5 spears)	*2 net carbs*
Beans, green, fresh	*3 net carbs*
Bean sprouts	*2 net carbs*
Bok choy	*.2 net carbs*
Broccoli, fresh	*2 net carbs*

Cabbage, all kinds	*1.5 net carbs*
Cauliflower	*1.5 net carbs*
Celery (2 stalks)	*1.5 net carbs*
Chard, Swiss	*1.5 net carbs*
Chayote squash	*2 net carbs*
Collard greens	*2 net carbs*
Cucumber	*1 net carbs*
Eggplant	*2 net carbs*
Fennel	*2 net carbs*
Garlic (1 clove)	*1 net carb*
Jicama	*2.5 net carbs*
Lettuce	*.5 net carbs*
Mushrooms	*2 net carbs*
Okra	*3 net carbs*
Onions	*5 net carbs*
Peppers, red or green bell	*3 net carbs*
Pumpkin meat	*4 net carbs*
Radicchio	*1 net carb*
Radishes	*1 net carb*
Scallions	*2.5 net carbs*
Snow peas	*3.4 net carbs*
Spinach, fresh	*.3 net carbs*
Spinach, frozen	*2 net carbs*
Squash, spaghetti	*4 net carbs*
Squash, yellow	*1.5 net carbs*
Squash, zucchini	*1.5 net carbs*
Tofu	*2.5 net carbs*
Tomato (1 small)	*3 net carbs*
Turnip	*2.5 net carbs*
Turnip greens	*1 net carb*
Watercress	*0 net carbs*

As you can see from your grocery list, there is no lack of food variety. What there is a lack of is pre-made, processed foods and SUGAR. With the above list, you can mix and match tons of recipes of good, fresh food low in SUGAR and high in vitamins and minerals. Yes, it requires you to cook and to prepare food. So what? I'm going to make it easy for you by providing you with lots of personal recipes. (I did mention I was a cook, didn't I? Yes, I'm quite sure I did. ☺)

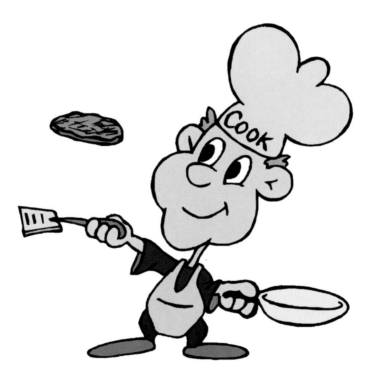

RECIPES
Snack Trays

Snack trays are by far the easiest way to fulfill your snacking needs. They offer a wide variety of choices and should be spun out of the previous night's entrée on a continual basis. If you don't want to cook and instead choose the eat-out options, you can still have snack trays. Most supermarkets and delis have, or can prepare, any kind of tray you want. Veggie trays, meat trays, cheese trays, and chicken-wing trays are all very common.

Chicken Pinwheels

INGREDIENTS
Sliced ham
Sliced Swiss cheese
Boneless chicken breast
Salt & pepper to taste

Lay out a thin slice of ham. Place a slice of Swiss cheese on top of the slice of ham and roll up. Using a sharp knife, cut a pocket inside of a boneless chicken breast. Stuff the rolled ham and cheese into the pocket and close with a wooden toothpick. Bake in preheated 375°F oven for 35 minutes. Let cool completely in fridge. Once cooled, using a sharp knife, slice the entire breast into ½-inch thick pinwheels. Arrange pinwheels on a tray and allow them to come to room temperature before serving.

TIP—Slice pinwheels from the extra chicken cordon bleu you made and refrigerated the evening before.

Chicken Wings

INGREDIENTS
Frozen chicken wings
Salt
Cayenne pepper
Walden Farms BBQ sauce

Buy the uncoated wings in your freezer section. Spice them up with salt and cayenne pepper or coat them with Walden Farms BBQ sauce.

Prosciutto, Provolone, and Asparagus Rollups

INGREDIENTS
Prosciutto sliced Italian ham
Provolone cheese
Asparagus
Extra virgin olive oil
Cracked black pepper
Romano cheese, ground
Salt

Buy thinly sliced prosciutto (salt-cured Italian ham) and provolone cheese from your local deli. Cook asparagus in a little salted water until cooked (but not mushy), cool asparagus in cold water, and pat dry. Lay out ham and place cheese on top, place a half stalk of asparagus inside, and roll up. When you have made as many as you like, sprinkle each one with extra virgin olive oil, a few grinds of cracked black pepper, and top with a sprinkling of ground Romano cheese. Let rest at room temperature for 20 minutes before serving.

Veggie Tray

INGREDIENTS
Broccoli florets
Cauliflower florets
Celery
Red bell pepper
Green beans
Zucchini squash
Hidden Valley Ranch Dressing
Salt

Cut up all the veggies into finger food sizes. Blanch the broccoli and cauliflower florets in boiling salted water for 60 seconds. Immediately cool the florets by submersing them in ice water to stop the cooking process. Drain and pat dry the florets before arranging on serving platter. You can use this list or any mix of veggies from the approved list. Serve with 2 or 3 low-SUGAR salad dressings for dips.

TIP—When you're chopping veggies, cut up plenty of extra and bag them up in the fridge for quick, easy replacement.

Celery with Cream Cheese & Chopped Green Olives

INGREDIENTS
Pitted green olives
Cream cheese
Celery
Ground black pepper

Mix chopped green olives with cream cheese, stuff the celery, and grind a little black pepper on top. Keep refrigerated.

Cheese and Crackers

INGREDIENTS
GG Bran CrispBread
Cream cheese
Scallions
Bacon bits
Block cheddar cheese
Block smoked Gouda
Block pepper Jack
Block Havarti

Use your GG Bran CrispBread as crackers. Slice a variety of cheeses, such as block cheddars, smoked Gouda, pepper Jack and Havarti, arrange on serving tray. Pan-fry a few strips of bacon until crisp. Finely chop the bacon strips and a couple of scallions and mix well with cream cheese. Place spread into serving bowl and center the bowl in the middle of the serving tray.

Genoa Salami Rolls Stuffed with Farmer's Cheese and Roasted Garlic Spread

INGREDIENTS
Head of garlic
Olive oil
Block of farmer's cheese
Mayonnaise
Genoa salami, sliced
Green olives, pitted
Toothpicks

Cut the top ¼ inch off a head of garlic, place in an oven-safe dish, and drizzle a tablespoon of olive oil over the head. Bake garlic at 350°F for 20 to 25 minutes, or until soft when squeezed. Crumble one 8 oz package of farmer's cheese into a mixing bowl and add 1 to 2 tablespoons of mayonnaise. When the garlic cools, squeeze all the cloves into the cheese and mix well. Place a teaspoon of filling into each piece of salami and roll it up. Stab a green olive with a toothpick and stick it into the roll. Arrange on serving tray and serve.

Cream Cheese and Lox Rollups

INGREDIENTS
Cream cheese
Capers
Lox (salt-cured salmon)
GG Bran CrispBread

Buy thinly sliced lox (salt-cured salmon) from your local market and lay out each slice individually. Spread a layer of whipped or fork-softened cream cheese on each slice, sprinkle capers on top of the cheese, and roll up your slices. Place toothpicks through each slice to make bite-size portions and slice with a sharp knife. Lay out on snack tray and serve with GG Bran CrispBread.

Deli Rollups

INGREDIENTS
Sliced deli turkey breast
Sliced deli ham
Sliced deli roast beef
Sliced deli Cuban pork
Sliced deli Munster cheese
Sliced deli American cheese
Sliced deli Swiss cheese
Sugar-free pickles
Hearts of palm
Asparagus
Broccoli stalks
Pitted green olives
Variety of mustards
Toothpicks

Buy thinly sliced meats and cheeses from your local deli.

Cook asparagus and broccoli stalks in a little salted water until cooked (but not mushy), cool vegetables in cold water, and pat dry. Lay out a variety of meat slices and place a variety of cheese slices on top, 1 slice of cheese per 1 slice of meat. Place a half stalk of asparagus inside, and roll up. Next one place a sliver of broccoli stalks inside and roll up. Next one place a sliver of heart of palm and roll up. Next one use a sliver of pickle and roll up. Place an olive through a toothpick and the toothpick through the rollups. Repeat the process. When you have made as many as you like, sprinkle each one with extra virgin olive oil, a few grinds of cracked black pepper, and top with a sprinkling of ground Romano cheese. Let rest at room temperature for 20 minutes before serving. Serve with a variety of mustards.

Deviled Eggs

INGREDIENTS
Jumbo eggs
Ice cubes
Mayonnaise
Dry mustard
Salt & pepper
Paprika

Place eggs in saucepan in a single layer, cover with enough cold water to be 2 inches above the shells. Cover the pot and bring to a boil over medium heat. As soon as the water starts to boil, remove pan from heat and let the eggs stand in hot water for 16 minutes. Drain off hot water and cover with cold water and some ice cubes. Let stand until eggs are completely cooled. Peel eggs under running water and pat dry. Slice eggs in half lengthwise and remove cooked yolks. Place yolks in mixing bowl and arrange sliced eggs onto serving platter. To the yolks, add mayonnaise, salt, pepper, and a little dry mustard. Mix the yolks until smooth and spoon back into the eggs. Sprinkle with paprika and refrigerate.

Beef Jerky

INGREDIENTS
London Broil (4 pounds)
Soy sauce
Worcestershire sauce
Liquid smoke
Sugar-free Teriyaki sauce
Splenda
Cajun Land Cajun seasoning

Slice 4 pounds of 1½–2-inch thick London broil steaks into 1/8-inch strips. Place strips in marinade for 48 hours *mixing well* halfway through the process. Drain marinade and place strips in food dehydrator, grind black pepper onto strips, and dehydrate per manufacturer's instructions.

Marinade—½ cup soy sauce, ¼ cup Worcestershire sauce, ¼ cup liquid smoke, ¼ cup teriyaki sauce, 2 tablespoons Splenda, 2 tablespoons Cajun Land Cajun seasoning.

WEB-FEATURE RECIPE!—Instructional video at http://www.fattoskinny.com Click the Recipes button.

BREAKFASTS

Corned Beef Hash and Eggs

INGREDIENTS
Jumbo eggs
Corned beef
Salt & pepper
GG Bran CrispBread

Use leftover corned beef from a corned beef dinner, chopped finely or open a can of corned beef. You can buy different brands at the store. Check the labels for carbs. Usually "hash" has potatoes, so stay with the can that says "corned beef." Put the contents into a covered, nonstick frying pan and heat on medium heat until hot. Hollow out 2 craters in the corned beef and drop an egg into each crater. Cover pan and lower heat to med/low. Cook for 3–5 minutes or until the 2 eggs develop an opaque look on top. Serve with GG Bran CrispBread.

TIP Plan on having this breakfast the morning after your corned beef and cabbage dinner.

Ham and Cheese Egg Beater Omelets with Sour Cream and Salsa

INGREDIENTS
Egg Beaters
Butter
Sour cream
Chopped ham
Cheddar cheese
Salsa
Salt & pepper
GG Bran CrispBread

Use Egg Beaters or another egg white, yolk-free product for this omelet. Over med/low heat, melt tab of butter in covered nonstick skillet. Beat 2 tablespoons of sour cream into ½ cup of egg product. Pour eggs into skillet and cover. Once egg starts to set, top with chopped ham and grated cheddar cheese and cover. Once egg is completely set, fold omelet in half and slip out of pan onto plate. Spoon on 2 tablespoons of salsa and top with a teaspoon of sour cream. Serve with GG Bran CrispBread.

TIP—Plan on having this breakfast the morning after your baked ham dinner.

Strawberry Pancakes and Bacon

INGREDIENTS
Eggs
Oil
New Hope Mills Low Carb Sugar Free Pancake & Waffle Mix
Butter
Strawberries
Log Cabin Sugar Free Syrup
Bacon

Prepare pancake mix as directed on the box. Add ¼ cup chopped fresh or thawed frozen strawberries to batter and cook over hot griddle. Serve with Louis Rich Turkey Bacon or pork bacon and Log Cabin Sugar-free Syrup.

TIP—Extra pancakes can be frozen or refrigerated. Heat them using a toaster oven. *Limit to once per week.*

Philly Cheesesteak and Egg Wraps

INGREDIENTS
Eggs
Sliced steak
Olive oil
Mozzarella cheese
Romaine lettuce leaf or La Tortilla Factory tortilla
Salt & pepper

Heat 2 tablespoons of olive oil in a nonstick skillet and brown thinly sliced steak and some thinly sliced onion, pushed to one side of skillet. Scramble an egg in the pan, then mix the egg with the meat. Throw in ¼ cup of shredded mozzarella cheese and toss around to mix. Drop a serving into a large romaine lettuce leaf, salt & pepper and roll up the wrap. If you prefer, you can substitute La Tortilla Factory tortillas for the romaine lettuce leaf. I prefer the greens as wraps to keep the meal 100% SUGAR-free.

TIP—When slicing up steak for meat on a stick, slice extra and freeze in individual portion sizes for this meal.

Mexican Omelet

INGREDIENTS
Eggs
Ground beef
Cheddar cheese
Sour cream
Salsa (low-sugar)
Olive oil
Cumin
Cayenne pepper
Salt & pepper

Pan-fry ground beef in olive oil and spice up with salt, pepper, cumin, and cayenne. Strain and set aside. Melt a tab of butter in a nonstick skillet over medium heat. Pour 2 well-beaten eggs into pan and cover. When eggs start to set, spoon in meat and cover with cheddar cheese, fold omelet, cover pan, and remove from heat. Leave covered 2 to 3 minutes, allowing cheese to melt. Slide omelet onto dish, spoon a couple of tablespoons of low-SUGAR salsa on top of omelet, place dollop of sour cream on top, and serve.

TIP—Wonderful light dinner or lunch, serve with avocado.

Breakfast Pepperoni and Cheese Pizza

INGREDIENTS
Egg Beaters
Sliced pepperoni
Jicama
Olive oil
Cheddar or mozzarella cheese
Parmesan or Romano grated cheese
Salt & pepper to taste

Preheat your oven to 350°F. Heat up 2 tablespoons of olive oil in an ovenproof skillet on stovetop at medium heat. Line the skillet with thin slices of jicama for your crust. Cook sliced jicama for 5 minutes in skillet. Add enough Egg Beaters or other egg product to cover crust ½-inch thick. Sprinkle ½–¾ cup shredded cheddar or mozzarella cheese on top of the eggs, place pepperoni generously on top, and move pan to oven. Bake for 25 minutes or until eggs are set. To check egg set, gently press center of pizza. If firm to the touch, eggs are set. Slice into pizza slices and sprinkle Parmesan or Romano cheese on top prior to serving.

TIP—To spice it up a bit, add chopped jalapeño peppers to the eggs. Works well at room temperature. Make an extra pizza and cube it up on a snack tray.

Berry Berry Pecan Waffles with Ham

INGREDIENTS
Eggs
Oil
Chopped pecans
New Hope Mills Low Carb Sugar Free Pancake & Waffle Mix
Butter
Fresh blackberries & raspberries
Log Cabin Sugar Free Syrup
Ham

Prepare waffle mix as directed on the box. Add ¼ cup chopped pecans to batter and cook per waffle maker instructions. Place a few fresh blackberries and raspberries on each waffle and top with Log Cabin Sugar Free Syrup. Serve with a slice of ham from ham night.

TIP—Extra waffles can be frozen or refrigerated. Heat them using a toaster oven. Limit to once per week.

Crepes Florentine

INGREDIENTS
Eggs
New Hope Mills Low Carb Sugar Free Pancake & Waffle Mix
Butter
Diced onion
Chopped frozen spinach
Bertolli Alfredo sauce

Crepes are very easy to make. They are simply very thin pancakes used to roll up a variety of ingredients. Preheat an 8-inch nonstick skillet over medium heat. Using a stick of butter, make sure the bottom of the pan and an inch or 2 up the sides is greased. Pour in a small amount of batter and, using the pan's handle, lift and swirl the pan to spread the batter out thinly across the entire bottom of the pan. Cover pan for 60 seconds. Crepe should be set on top and can now be gently removed from pan onto a plate. Repeat the process, stacking the crepes on top of one another and separated with paper towels until you have made all the crepes you need. Place the filling into each crepe and roll them up. Top with sauce when served.

Batter—One tablespoon of New Hope Mills Low Carb Sugar Free Pancake & Waffle Mix, 1 egg, 1 teaspoon water. Makes two 8-inch crepes.

Filling—Using the same skillet, sauté in butter a tablespoon of diced onion, until soft, add 1 cup of chopped spinach (previously frozen) and ¼ cup of Alfredo sauce. Put a couple of heaping tablespoons of filling into each crepe and roll up, top with little more Alfredo sauce.

Sauce—Bertolli Alfredo sauce

TIP—Make extra crepes and leave in the fridge between paper towels for a dessert tonight. Fill with chopped strawberries and top with Reddi-wip for strawberry shortcake crepe.

Crabmeat Omelet Alfredo

INGREDIENTS
Egg Beaters
Diced onion
Diced bell pepper
Diced garlic
Crabmeat (canned)
Butter
Bertolli Alfredo sauce
Salt & pepper to taste

In a skillet, sauté in butter a tablespoon of diced onion, a tablespoon of diced bell pepper, and a diced garlic clove until soft. Add 1 small can of crabmeat and 2 or 3 tablespoons of Alfredo sauce. Set filling aside. Wipe out your skillet and add a teaspoon of butter to melt on medium heat. Pour in ½ cup of Egg Beaters and cover. When egg sets on top, pour in filling and fold over. Serve with a small amount of sauce on top.

Sauce—Bertolli Alfredo sauce

Lox and Cream Cheese with Capers and Red Onion

INGREDIENTS
Cream cheese
Capers
Chopped red onion
Lox (salt-cured salmon)
Ground black pepper
GG Bran CrispBread

Lox or gravlox is thinly sliced salt-cured salmon found in your grocer's seafood section. Spread Philly (plain or salmon flavored) cream cheese onto GG Bran CrispBread. Sprinkle capers and chopped red onion onto cream cheese and top with a slice of lox. Grind some black pepper on top and serve.

The Western

INGREDIENTS
Egg Beaters
Chopped onion
Chopped green, yellow and red bell pepper
Butter
Salt & pepper

Melt a teaspoon of butter in a nonstick omelet skillet over medium heat. Sauté ¼ cup of onion, along with a ½ cup of the chopped bell pepper mix for 2 minutes. Add ½ cup of Egg Beaters and gently combine the ingredients. Cover and cook for 2 minutes, flip the western and cook another minute. Serve immediately with a low-SUGAR salsa.

TIP—You can sprinkle grated Italian or cheddar cheese on top of your western during the last minute of cooking for an interesting variation.

LUNCHES

Tuna Wrap with Black Olives and Jalapeño

INGREDIENTS
Tuna (canned)
Black olives
Jalapeño pepper
Mayonnaise
Romaine lettuce or La Tortilla Factory tortillas
Fried pork skins
Dill pickle

Salt & pepper

Make your tuna with your favorite mayonnaise. Add chopped black olives and chopped jalapeño pepper. Place in a large romaine lettuce leaf, salt & pepper, and roll up wrap. If you prefer, you can substitute La Tortilla Factory tortillas for the romaine lettuce leaf. I prefer the greens as wraps to keep the meal 100% SUGAR-free. Serve with fried pork skins and a dill pickle.

TIP—Wraps can be made from the leftovers in your fridge or from the wide variety of meats and cheeses available from your deli. When buying sliced lunchmeat, make sure to stay away from any meats cured with SUGAR or honey. CHECK THE LABELS.

Italian Chef's Salad with Radicchio and Walnuts

INGREDIENTS
Mixed lettuces
Radicchio
Italian ham (prosciutto)
Genoa salami
Mortadella
Provolone cheese
Green olives, pitted
Hard-boiled egg
Chopped walnuts
Red wine vinegar
Extra virgin olive oil

Prepare bed of your favorite lettuces, including radicchio in the mix. Roll up slices of Italian ham, Genoa salami, mortadella, and provolone cheese and place on greens. Add some green olives and a hard-boiled egg, cut in half. Sprinkle chopped walnuts on top. Serve with red wine vinegar and olive oil as a dressing.

TIP—While you have the greens out, prepare some side salads in bowls that you can leave covered with plastic wrap in the fridge. While the meat and cheese are out, do some rollups for a snack tray.

Deep-fried Shrimp with Sweet and Hot Wasabi Jicama Coleslaw

INGREDIENTS
Green cabbage
Purple cabbage
Jicama
Wasabi mustard (mixed from powder or in tube)
Kraft Green Goddess dressing
Sour cream
Mayonnaise
Stevia sweetener
Shrimp
Eggs
Unflavored fried pork skins
Sugar-free catsup
Prepared horseradish
Salt & pepper

Slice ½ green cabbage and ¼ purple cabbage into thin slices. Rough chop and place in mixing bowl. Peel and slice ½ medium jicama into thin slices, then julienne and rough chop, place in mixing bowl. Salt and pepper vegetables. In a separate bowl, mix 1 tablespoon wasabi mustard (mixed from powder or in tube), 3 tablespoons Kraft Green Goddess dressing, 1 tablespoon sour cream, 1 tablespoon mayonnaise, and 1 teaspoon powdered stevia sweetener. Add dressing to cabbage and jicama and mix well, let stand. Clean and de-vein shrimp, place in egg wash. Process unflavored pork rinds in food processor until finely ground. Using the pork rind "flour," coat shrimp and deep fry until golden brown. Serve shrimp with cocktail sauce made with SUGAR-free catsup and horseradish.

TIP—Process extra pork rinds in food processor and store ground, deep-fry coating in a ziplock bag in the pantry. Coating works well for all fried foods, including fish and chicken. Coleslaw is very good the next day, too, if you wish to make a double batch.

Grilled Cheeseburger and Chips

INGREDIENTS
Ground beef
Favorite burger cheese
Sliced onion
Sliced tomato
Romaine lettuce or La Tortilla Factory tortillas
Pork rinds or EatSmart Soy Crisps
Dill pickles (sugar-free)

Grill that burger any way you like it, top with your favorite cheese (try smoked Gouda for a change) and cut in half. Serve burger in a large romaine lettuce leaf with onion and tomato. If you prefer, you can substitute La Tortilla Factory tortillas for the romaine lettuce leaf. I prefer the greens as wraps to keep the burger 100% SUGAR-free. Serve with pork rinds or a measured amount of EatSmart Soy Crisps and a big dill pickle (SUGAR-free, of course).

Mexican Taco Salad

INGREDIENTS
Ground beef
Favorite salad mix
Chopped onion
Chopped garlic
Chopped jalapeño pepper
Cumin
Salt & pepper to taste
Olive oil
EatSmart Soy Crisps
Cheddar cheese

Heat up a tablespoon of olive oil in a skillet. Pan-fry ground beef with onions, garlic, salt & pepper, chopped jalapeño pepper, and cumin. Drain meat in strainer. Place EatSmart Soy Crisps around the rim of a bowl filled with of your favorite salad mix. Spoon a generous amount of meat on top while still hot and sprinkle with grated cheddar cheese. Serve immediately.

TIP—Plan this lunch the day after your cheeseburgers to use up the ground beef in the fridge.

Jamaican Jerk Chicken with Strawberry Sauce

INGREDIENTS
Boneless chicken breasts
Jamaican jerk seasoning
Strawberries
Ice
Lettuce
Salt & pepper to taste

Heat up grill, using a sharp knife, make several deep cuts into the boneless breasts. Rub breasts with dry or wet Jamaican jerk seasoning. Check the label for SUGAR. My personal favorite is Walkerswood brand; it's most likely at your supermarket or at **www.walkerswood.com**. Place breasts on hot grill. While the chicken is grilling, put some strawberries in your blender with a little ice and hit the switch. Arrange a bed of lettuce on a plate and pour a generous amount of strawberry sauce in the middle, reserving a few tablespoons for a topping. Slice each breast on an angle and fan across sauce, decorate the top with the reserved sauce, and serve.

TIP—Cook extra breasts for a snack tray, cut in strips, and serve at room temperature. Dip into cold strawberry sauce.

Steak and Chicken Fajitas with Spicy Avocado Spread

INGREDIENTS
Steak
Boneless chicken breast
Sliced onion
Sliced bell pepper
Cumin
Ground red pepper
Salt & pepper to taste
Olive oil
Romaine lettuce or La Tortilla Factory tortillas
Hass avocado
Sour cream
Cheddar cheese

Prepare steak and chicken by cutting into thin strips, season meat with salt, pepper, and cumin, and set aside. Cut an appropriate amount of onion & bell pepper into thin strips, season with salt, pepper, and cumin, set aside. Using a Hass avocado, scoop the fruit into a bowl, add 1 tablespoon of sour cream and ¼ teaspoon ground red pepper to each ¼ cup of fruit, mash fruit into paste, and salt and pepper to taste. Heat a tablespoon of olive oil in a cast iron skillet on high heat. When oil begins to smoke, quickly stir-fry all ingredients until chicken is cooked through. Place steaming hot skillet on trivet in the center of your table. Arrange a plate of large romaine lettuce leaves to be used as a wrap. If you prefer, you can substitute La Tortilla Factory tortillas for the romaine lettuce leaf. I prefer the greens as wraps to keep the meal 100% SUGAR-free. Serve with shredded cheddar cheese, sour cream and avocado spread.

TIP—Cook extra for salad toppings.

Fajita Salad

Using the recipe above, omit the avocado spread and serve the meat and vegetables on top of a green salad. Serve each guest ½ Hass avocado with 1 tablespoon of sour cream in seed cavity and a squirt of lemon on top as a side dish.

Stir Fry Surprise

INGREDIENTS
Leftover cooked protein
(such as shrimp, chicken, beef, pork, turkey, or fish)
Diced garlic
Diced ginger
Olive oil
Sliced onion
Sliced bell pepper
Chopped cabbage
Chopped bok choy
Snow pea pods
Mushrooms
Bean sprouts
Soy sauce (low-sugar)

This is a fast, easy meal. Heat 2 tablespoons of olive oil on high heat. When oil starts to smoke, add 1 teaspoon each of chopped fresh garlic and ginger. Immediately add a mixture of chopped green cabbage, bok choy, snow pea pods, mushrooms, onion, bean sprouts, bell pepper, and low-SUGAR soy sauce in measured amounts and stir-fry. Add leftover cooked protein (such as shrimp, chicken, beef, pork, turkey, or fish) to vegetables and cook until heated through or omit protein and serve as a vegetable dish.

TIP—While you're chopping the veggies, chop enough to have a bag full of mixed stir-fry in the fridge for quick meals.

Chicken Pecan Salad

INGREDIENTS
Leftover cooked chicken
Chopped green or purple onion
Rough chopped pecans
Mayonnaise
Favorite green salad mix
Salt & pepper to taste

This is an easy recipe to make after any baked chicken meal. In a bowl combine leftover chicken chopped into small chunks, some chopped green or purple onion, a couple of tablespoons of pecans and enough mayonnaise to dampen to your liking. Salt and pepper salad to your individual taste and serve. This salad can be served inside a wrap or simply scoop on top of your favorite green salad mix.

Cajun Seafood Salad

INGREDIENTS
Leftover Cajun fish & shrimp
Chopped green or purple onion
Mayonnaise
Salt & pepper to taste

I make this wonderful salad the day after we have a Cajun seafood boil (recipe in dinner section). Chop leftover fish and shrimp from the boil and place into a mixing bowl. Add chopped green or purple onion and mayonnaise to taste mix well. Salt & pepper to taste, and serve. This is best served over a green salad or as a wrap in La Tortilla

Factory tortillas or a romaine lettuce leaf. You can also serve as a spread using GG Bran CrispBread.

TIP—You can substitute canned tuna by simply spicing up the tuna with Cajun Land Cajun seasoning.

Italian Sausage, Onion, and Pepper Wraps

INGREDIENTS
Olive oil
Italian sausage
Sliced onion
Sliced bell pepper
Romaine lettuce or La Tortilla Factory tortillas
Salt & pepper to taste

Heat 1 tablespoon of olive oil in skillet at medium heat. Brown sausage until cooked through. Rough chop or slice green bell pepper and onion, add to the pan, and cover. Cook until vegetables soften. Serve in large romaine lettuce leaves used as a wrap. If you prefer, you can substitute La Tortilla Factory tortillas for the romaine lettuce leaf, but I prefer the greens as wraps to keep the meal 100% SUGAR-free.

TIP—Cook extra sausages and cut them into 1-inch pieces. Stick a toothpick in each one and place in fridge for a snack tray. Reheat gently in microwave before serving, using leftover sauce for dip.

Crab Cakes

INGREDIENTS
Eggs
Olive oil
Lump crabmeat
New Hope Mills Low Carb Sugar Free Pancake & Waffle Mix
Chopped green bell pepper
Chopped onion
Unflavored pork rinds
Salt & pepper to taste
Hot sauce

Buy a can of pasteurized lump crabmeat from your grocer's seafood department. In a mixing bowl, combine 1 cup of crab, 1 egg, ¼ cup chopped onion, ¼ cup chopped green pepper, 2 tablespoons ground pork rinds, and 2 tablespoons New Hope Mills Low Carb Sugar Free Pancake & Waffle Mix. Mix gently as to not break up the crab too much. Heat 2 tablespoons of olive oil in nonstick skillet on med/high heat. Mold small patties and drop into hot oil, flip when edges get light brown, salt and pepper, and serve with hot sauce.

Zucchini Alfredo

INGREDIENTS
Olive oil
Zucchini squash
Bertolli Alfredo sauce
Ground Parmesan or Romano cheese
Ground black pepper
Salt to taste

Julianne zucchini lengthwise, quickly sauté in hot olive oil, add Bertolli Alfredo sauce to coat, serve immediately. Grind fresh Parmesan or Romano cheese and black pepper on top, salt to taste.

Baked Mushroom Caps with Crabmeat Stuffing

INGREDIENTS
Lump crabmeat
Egg
Chopped onion
Chopped green bell pepper
Cheddar cheese
Large mushroom caps
Hot sauce
Salt & pepper to taste

Buy a can of pasteurized lump crabmeat from your grocer's seafood department. In a mixing bowl, combine 1 cup of crab, 1 egg, ¼ cup chopped onion, ¼ cup chopped green pepper, and ¼ cup shredded cheddar cheese. Place large mushroom caps on a cookie sheet. Stuff each cap and bake at 425°F for 10–12 minutes. Serve with hot sauce.

TIP—Substitute artichoke hearts for the mushroom caps for Baked Artichoke Hearts with Crabmeat Stuffing.

Cajun Boiled Shrimp

INGREDIENTS
Large raw shrimp
Cajun Land Cajun seasoning
Butter
Green salad

Bring 1 quart of water to a boil, adding 1 heaping tablespoon of Cajun Land Cajun seasoning to the water. Place 1 or 2 pounds of shrimp into the water and cook until pink—*do not overcook*. Strain and serve with melted butter and a green salad.

Egg Fu Yung

INGREDIENTS
Olive oil
Eggs
Bean sprouts
Chopped scallions
Diced cooked chicken or ham
Heinz Classic Chicken Gravy
Salt & pepper to taste

In a mixing bowl, beat 4 eggs or use egg substitute. To the eggs, add 1 can of bean sprouts well drained, ½ cup of chopped scallions, and ½ cup of diced, cooked chicken or ham. Mix well. Heat 1 tablespoon of olive oil in a nonstick skillet at medium heat. Cook your Egg Fu Yung pancakes in covered skillet, flipping once. Serve immediately topped with Heinz Classic Chicken Gravy.

Macafoney and Cheese

INGREDIENTS
Extra firm tofu
Shredded cheddar cheese
Bertolli Alfredo sauce
Eggs
Chopped onion
Cubed cooked ham if desired
Ground Parmesan or Romano cheese
Salt & pepper to taste

Preheat oven to 375°F. In a mixing bowl, combine 1 pound tofu (extra firm, well-drained, and cubed into ½-inch cubes), 2 cups cheddar cheese, 2 eggs, beaten, 1/3 cup Bertolli Alfredo sauce, and salt and pepper. If desired, cubed ham can also be added. Pour mixture into a well-greased, shallow casserole dish, individual casseroles, or pie plate. Bake at 375°F for 30–45 minutes until golden brown and slightly crunchy on top. Sprinkle grated Parmesan or Romano cheese on top prior to serving.

COOKING TIP—Cook this recipe in individual baking dishes, prepare extras, and freeze uncooked inside individual bakeware for a fast, easy meal.

WEB-FEATURE RECIPE!—Instructional video at http://www.fattoskinny.com Click the Recipes button.

Ham and Cheese Soufflé

INGREDIENTS
Shredded cheddar cheese
Bertolli Alfredo sauce
Eggs
Butter
Cream of tartar
Diced onion
Diced cooked ham
Salt & pepper to taste

Preheat oven to 375°F. Well grease 2 small or 1 medium soufflé dish with butter, set aside. In 2 mixing bowls separate 6 eggs, whites in one bowl and yolks in another. Beat the yolks until they are a light yellow color, add ¾ cup of shredded cheddar cheese, ¾ cup diced ham, and ½ cup diced onion, mix well and set aside. Add a pinch of cream of tartar to the egg whites and beat until they are stiff. Using a baking spatula scoop out 1/3 of the beaten egg whites and fold them into the egg yolk mixture to lighten it up. Now fold the egg yolk mixture into the remaining egg whites, being careful not to over mix. The finished mixture should be light and fluffy. Gently transfer the mixture into your soufflé dish or dishes and place in oven for 30 minutes. While the soufflé is cooking heat up 1 cup of Bertolli Alfredo Sauce and melt ¼ cup of shredded cheddar cheese into sauce. Serve as sauce for soufflé. Serve your soufflé with a side green salad and GG Bran CrispBread.

TIP—Don't be afraid of soufflés! They are very easy to make and make wonderful lunches, breakfasts, or even dinners and deserts. Get creative by replacing the ham with well-drained chopped frozen spinach brought to room temp. Try using a couple of packages of Swiss Miss Sensible Sweets Diet 25 Calorie Cocoa Mix instead of ham and cheese to make a chocolate soufflé. Crabmeat or chopped shrimp make a wonderful seafood soufflé. The possibilities are endless.

DINNERS

Baked Ham with Beans and Potatoes

INGREDIENTS
Olive oil
Ham
Cauliflower
Mayonnaise
Benecol spread or butter
Pole beans
Diced garlic
Ground Parmesan or Romano cheese
Salt & pepper to taste

There are several hams on the market in your grocer's meat case. The average low-SUGAR ham ranges from 0 to 4 carbs per serving. Find the lowest. Bake the ham per the package instructions. Steam a head of cauliflower in a couple of inches of water until fork tender. Drain cauliflower and place into a food processor with a chopping blade. Add 2 tablespoons of your favorite mayonnaise, 1 tablespoon of Benecol spread or butter, and salt & pepper. Process until smooth. You now have your replacement mashed potatoes. Clean your pole beans and cut off the ends, steam until fork tender. Drain and leave in strainer. Return pot to stove and heat a couple of tablespoons of olive oil, sauté 2 or 3 cloves of diced garlic. When the garlic is cooked, return the beans to the pot and toss to coat. Add ¼ cup of grated Romano or Parmesan cheese and toss again. Transfer to serving plate. Serve Jell-O with Reddi-wip or Breyers CarbSmart ice cream for dessert.

TIP—Cut off a couple of thick slices of ham and cube them. Stick a green olive on a toothpick and stab the ham cube. Repeat until completed. Place in fridge for a snack tray.

Chicken Cordon Bleu and Broccoli with Lemon Butter

INGREDIENTS
Sliced ham
Swiss cheese
Boneless chicken breast
Butter
Head of broccoli
Lemon juice
Salt & pepper to taste

Slice off a thin slice of ham from your baked ham. Place a slice of Swiss cheese on top of the slice of ham and roll up. Using a sharp knife, cut a pocket inside of a boneless chicken breast. Stuff the rolled ham and cheese into the pocket and close with a wooden toothpick. Bake in preheated 375°F oven for 35 minutes. Steam a head of broccoli and serve with lemon butter. Prepare lemon butter by melting a ¼ stick of butter in microwave and adding 1 teaspoon of lemon juice to the butter.

TIP—Make a couple of extra chicken cordon bleus and place in fridge to cool. In the morning, slice the breasts into pinwheels and place on tray in fridge for snacks.

COOKING TIP—Cook this recipe in individual baking dishes, prepare extras, and freeze uncooked inside individual bakeware for a fast, easy dinner.

Corned Beef and Cabbage Boil with Onion and Green Beans

INGREDIENTS
Corned beef
Green cabbage
Onions
Green beans
Mustard

Buy a fresh corned beef from the grocer and boil per package instructions. When beef is done, add wedges of green cabbage and onions plus green beans to the water. Cook vegetables until desired tenderness. Serve with favorite mustard. Beef is done when it is fork tender.

TIP—Put remaining corned beef into food processor and chop for breakfast corned beef hash.

Cajun Seafood Boil

INGREDIENTS
Fish filets
Raw shrimp
Cajun Land Cajun seasoning
Green cabbage
Onions
Green beans
Cheesecloth & twist ties

In a large pot bring 2 quarts of water to a boil. Add 2 or 3 heaping tablespoons of Cajun Land Cajun seasoning to the water. Prepare white fish filets of your choice (I prefer grouper) by enclosing each filet in a cheesecloth wrap pulled into a sack and tied with a twist tie. Drop fish bags into the water along with wedges of green cabbage, onions cut in halves, and green beans. Boil for about 10 minutes then add fresh or frozen thawed out raw shrimp. Boil another 2 or 3 minutes or until shrimp is pink. Serve immediately.

TIP—Cook extra fish and shrimp to chop the next day for Cajun Seafood Salad.

Italian Stuffed Chicken Breast with Romano Green Beans

INGREDIENTS
Olive oil
Butter
Boneless chicken breast
Ricotta cheese
Shredded mozzarella cheese
Frozen chopped spinach
Low-sugar Italian pasta tomato sauce
Green beans
Diced garlic
Ground Romano cheese
Salt & pepper to taste

In a mixing bowl, combine 1 cup of ricotta cheese, ½ cup shredded mozzarella cheese, ½ cup previously frozen chopped spinach, salt and pepper to taste. Mix well and place into gallon ziplock bag. Using a sharp knife, cut a pocket inside of boneless chicken breasts. Cut a SMALL corner off your ziplock bag and pipe the filling into the pockets, close with a wooden toothpick. Place breasts into individual baking dishes, ladle some of your favorite low-SUGAR Italian pasta tomato sauce over breast, sprinkle a generous amount of shredded mozzarella cheese on top and bake in preheated 350°F oven for 30 minutes. Steam green beans to desired doneness, place into skillet with 1 tablespoon of butter, 1 tablespoon of extra virgin olive oil and 2 cloves of diced garlic. Sauté for 3–5 minutes, put on serving plate, and grate a generous amount of Romano cheese on top.

TIP—Make a couple of extras to cool. In the morning, slice the breasts into pinwheels and place on tray in fridge for snacks.

COOKING TIP—Cook this recipe in individual baking dishes, prepare extras, and freeze uncooked inside individual bakeware for a fast, easy dinner.

Shrimp Scampi on Spaghetti Squash

INGREDIENTS
Olive oil
Butter
Spaghetti squash
Large raw shrimp
Diced garlic
Ground Parmesan or Romano cheese
Salt & pepper to taste
Fresh spinach
Feta cheese
Olives

Punch some steam vent holes into your medium-size spaghetti squash with a sharp knife (10 or 12 will do, about 2 inches deep). Place spaghetti squash in microwave and cook on high heat for about 20 minutes. To test doneness, gently squeeze with a gloved hand. If the squash gives, then it's done. If not, cook at 5-minute intervals until soft enough to give when squeezed. When done, place on cutting board and cut in half lengthwise, let stand to cool. On medium, heat up 2 tablespoons of olive oil and 1 tablespoon of butter in skillet. Sauté 3 cloves of crushed garlic in skillet until signs of light brown appear. Add 2 pounds of cleaned, unfrozen shrimp to the skillet and sauté until shrimp become pink. Set skillet off heat. With a fork, remove seeds from squash and discard. Now, using the fork, start pulling out the squash meat onto a plate. Notice how the meat looks like strands of angel hair pasta. Salt & pepper the squash and toss with Romano or Parmesan cheese. Once the squash is "dressed," transfer portions to dinner plates and smother with your shrimp mixture. Serve with spinach salad topped with feta cheese and olives.

TIP—Cook extra shrimp for tomorrow's snack tray in fridge.

Roast Turkey with "Mashed Potatoes" and Baked Asparagus

INGREDIENTS
Olive oil
Butter
Turkey
Cauliflower
Mayonnaise
Asparagus
Ground Parmesan or Romano cheese
Salt & pepper to taste

Roast turkey per package instructions in roasting pan. Prepare "mashed potatoes" by steaming a head of cauliflower in a couple of inches of water until fork tender. Drain cauliflower and place into food processor with a chopping blade. Add 2 tablespoons of your favorite mayonnaise, 1 tablespoon of Benecol spread or butter, and salt & pepper. Process until smooth. Cut 1 inch off the bottoms of the asparagus and place in shallow baking dish. Brush all stalks with olive oil and salt & pepper. Bake for 20–30 minutes or until fork tender. Roll asparagus once in the baking dish to pick up the remaining olive oil and plate. Sprinkle grated Parmesan or Romano on top and pepper with a pepper grinder.

TIP—Buy a large enough turkey or turkey breast so you have plenty of leftovers for snack trays, lunchmeat, and chef's salad toppings.

BBQ Steak and Drumsticks with Grilled Vegetables

INGREDIENTS
Olive oil
Chicken drumsticks
Steak
Walden Farms BBQ sauce
Zucchini
Yellow squash
Bell pepper
Salt & pepper to taste

Preheat grill and BBQ chicken drumsticks. Use Walden Farms SUGAR-free BBQ sauce for chicken. When almost done, make sure there's room on the grill-top and grill your favorite steaks any way you like, but avoiding any marinades that contain SUGAR or carbs. Slice lengthwise zucchini and yellow squash into ½-inch thick slices. Slice bell pepper in half and flatten. Brush all vegetables with olive oil, salt and pepper each side, and grill.

TIP—Slice additional steaks into strips and freeze some of the strips in single servings for Philly cheesesteak wraps. Skewer the rest onto bamboo skewers, paint with soy sauce, and grill. Place in fridge along with leftover chicken drumsticks for snack trays.

Baked Salmon and Fennel in Parchment Paper with Sweet Lemon Caper Sauce

INGREDIENTS
Butter
Salmon
Fennel bulb
Capers
Splenda or stevia
Lemon juice
Salt & pepper to taste
Green salad

Place each piece of salmon in the middle of a 12-inch square piece of parchment paper, skin side down. Next to the fish, place a half fennel bulb. Salt & pepper and paint the fish and the fennel with butter. Loosely place another piece of parchment paper on top of the food and fold the 4 edges together to form a pouch, much like you would do if you were using aluminum foil. When your pouch is complete and sealed around all 4 edges, the top piece should be an inch or so above the food. Cut a small slit in the top piece to allow steam to escape. Place packages on a cookie sheet and bake in a preheated 350°F oven for 30 minutes. Melt a half stick of butter in the microwave. To the melted butter, add 1 tablespoon of capers, 1 teaspoon of Splenda or stevia, and 1 tablespoon of lemon juice. Spoon the sauce over the fish and fennel when served. Serve with a green salad on the side.

TIP—Cook an extra piece of fish and put in fridge to cool. Once cool, place skinless fish in food processor with a tablespoon or 2 of mayonnaise. Process until smooth, mix in finely chopped onion and capers, and salt & pepper for a wonderful salmon spread on GG Bran CrispBread.

Roast Cajun Pork Loin with Creamed Spinach Alfredo and Mushrooms

INGREDIENTS
Pork loin
Olive oil
Cajun Land Cajun seasoning
Frozen chopped spinach
Mushrooms
Diced garlic
Bertolli Alfredo sauce
Cheddar cheese
Salt & pepper to taste

Preheat oven to 375°F. Heat 2 tablespoons of olive oil on med/high heat. Score (in several places and ¼-inch deep) the fat side of a 2-pound pork loin roast with a sharp knife. Dry rub the entire roast with Cajun Land brand Cajun seasoning (**www.cajunlandbrand.com**). Braise all sides of the roast in the hot oil. Once braised, place skillet in the oven and roast for 40 minutes or until 130°F. In another skillet, heat up 1 box of frozen chopped spinach, ½ cup fresh chopped mushrooms, and ½ jar of Bertolli Alfredo sauce and a clove of diced garlic. Continue to cook on med/low heat until mushrooms are cooked through. Sprinkle ¼ cup of shredded cheddar cheese on top, cover, and remove from heat.

TIP—Make a double batch of spinach for Crepes Florentine filling.

Grouper Florentine with Baby Greens and Dill Dressing
(2 servings)

INGREDIENTS
Grouper filets
Butter
Frozen chopped spinach
Chopped onion
Diced garlic
Bertolli Alfredo sauce
Cooking sherry
Cheddar cheese
Salt & pepper to taste
Baby greens
Makoto brand dill dressing

Preheat oven to 400°F. Squeeze the water out of a box of frozen spinach and place spinach in mixing bowl. Rough chop ½ small onion and toss in bowl, add ½ jar of Bertolli Alfredo sauce, ¼ cup of cooking sherry, 2 cloves of diced garlic, ¼ cup of shredded cheddar cheese, and mix up the "goop." ☺ Split the goop between 2 individual baking dishes that have been well buttered. Place a nice filet of grouper into the goop and press down, flip the filet over and salt & pepper, top it with a couple of tabs of butter and bake for 25–30 minutes. Serve with baby greens from your produce dept and Makoto brand dill dressing (**www.makotodressing.com**).

TIP—You can use any fish of your choice, or even shrimp or a chicken breast. If you use a chicken breast, cook long enough for chicken to be cooked through. These freeze beautifully in individual baking dishes for quick dinners. I always make 4 at a time: 2 for us and 2 for the freezer.

Chicken Cacciatore with Spaghetti Squash
(2 servings)

INGREDIENTS
Olive oil
Boneless chicken breast
Spaghetti squash
Chopped onion
Chopped bell pepper
Chopped mushrooms
Diced garlic
Low-sugar Italian pasta tomato sauce
Ground Parmesan or Romano cheese
Salt & pepper to taste

Punch some steam vent holes into your medium-size spaghetti squash with a sharp knife (10 or 12 will do, about 2 inches deep). Place spaghetti squash in microwave and cook on high heat for about 20 minutes. To test doneness, gently squeeze with a gloved hand. If the squash gives, then it's done. If not, cook at 5-minute intervals until soft enough to give when squeezed. When done, place on cutting board and cut in half lengthwise, let stand to cool. Heat 2 tablespoons of olive oil in skillet on medium high heat. Pan-fry 1 cup of cubed chicken breast until nicely browned, remove chicken from pan, and set aside. To drippings, add 2 cloves of diced garlic, ½ cup chopped onions, ½ cup chopped bell pepper, and ½ cup mushrooms. Cook uncovered for 5 minutes.

Add 1 cup of your favorite low-SUGAR tomato sauce. When mixture comes back to heat, add chicken cover and reduce heat to simmer. After 5 minutes, remove from heat and let rest. With a fork, remove the seeds from the squash and discard. Now, using the fork, start pulling out the squash meat onto a plate. Notice how the meat looks like strands of angel hair pasta. Salt & pepper the squash and toss with Romano or Parmesan cheese. Once the squash is "dressed," transfer portions to dinner plates and smother with your cacciatore. Grind additional Romano or Parmesan cheese on top when serving.

TIP—You can substitute Italian sausage for sausage cacciatore. You can substitute Tofu Shirataki Pasta for the spaghetti squash.

Lasagna!

INGREDIENTS
Olive oil
Ground beef
Zucchini squash
Egg
Ricotta cheese
Mozzarella cheese
Diced garlic
Italian seasoning
Low-sugar Italian pasta tomato sauce
Ground Parmesan or Romano cheese
Salt & pepper to taste
Green salad

Preheat oven to 350°F. Heat 2 tablespoons of olive oil on medium heat, add 2 cloves of diced garlic and ½ pound of ground beef. Season beef with salt, pepper, and ½ teaspoon of Italian seasoning. Cook until done, drain fat, and set aside. In a mixing bowl, combine 1 egg, 1 cup of ricotta cheese, and ½ cup shredded mozzarella cheese. Salt and pepper to taste, mix well, and set aside. Cut very thin strips of zucchini squash lengthwise to take the place of lasagna noodles. Put a couple of tablespoons of your favorite low-SUGAR tomato sauce into the bottoms of 2 individual baking dishes and add a couple of squash slices. Spoon on half of the cheese mixture as the next layer, sprinkle with a little more sauce, and place in a couple of squash slices as your next layer. Next, place a layer of meat, then a little more sauce, lay in a couple more squash slices, topping it all with more sauce. Sprinkle desired amount of shredded mozzarella cheese on top and bake for 30 minutes. Serve with green salad.

TIP—You can substitute Italian sausage or any ground meats (even a mixture of several) for the ground beef. These freeze beautifully in individual baking dishes for quick dinners. I always make 4 at a time: 2 for us and 2 for the freezer.

COOKING TIP—Cook this recipe in individual baking dishes, prepare extras, and freeze uncooked portions inside individual bakeware for a fast, easy dinner.

Seafood Bake

INGREDIENTS
Butter
Scallops
Shrimp
Fish
Garlic salt
Ground pepper
Paprika

Buy scallops, shrimp, and your choice of fish from your local seafood market. (If you can't get fresh, frozen works well.) In the microwave, melt a tablespoon of butter in each individual baking dish, then place a portion of each seafood in the dish and roll around in the butter to coat each side. Arrange neatly in the dish and sprinkle with garlic salt, ground pepper, and paprika. Bake in a 425°F oven for 15 minutes, or until seafood is cooked through.

COOKING TIP—Cook this recipe in individual baking dishes, prepare extras, and freeze uncooked portions inside individual bakeware for a fast, easy dinner.

Shepherd's Pie

INGREDIENTS
Olive oil
Ground beef
Chopped onion
Ricotta cheese
Shredded cheddar cheese
Shredded mozzarella cheese
Cauliflower
Butter
Mayonnaise
Salt & pepper to taste

Heat 1 tablespoon of olive oil in a skillet. Brown ½ cup of chopped onions and ¾ pound of crumbled ground beef until cooked. Salt and pepper beef to taste and strain, and then set aside. In a mixing bowl, combine 1 cup of ricotta cheese, ½ cup of shredded cheddar cheese, and ½ cup of mozzarella cheese. Place ½ of the cooked ground beef and onions into a casserole dish. Layer, on top of the meat, ½ of the cheese, then cauliflower "mashed potatoes" (recipe below), then the remaining meat, and then cover all of it with a final layer: the remaining cheese. Bake uncovered in 350°F oven for 40–45 minutes.

Cauliflower "Mashed Potatoes"—Prepare "mashed potatoes" by steaming a head of cauliflower in a couple of inches of water until fork tender. Drain cauliflower and place into food processor with a chopping blade. Add 2 tablespoons of your favorite mayonnaise, 1 tablespoon of Benecol spread or butter, and salt & pepper. Process until smooth.

Veal Parmesan with Spaghetti Squash

INGREDIENTS
Olive oil
Veal cutlets
Zucchini squash
Egg wash (beaten egg with a little milk)
Ground pork rinds
Spaghetti squash
Mozzarella cheese
Low-sugar Italian pasta tomato sauce
Ground Parmesan or Romano cheese
Salt & pepper to taste
Green salad

Punch some steam vent holes into your medium-size spaghetti squash with a sharp knife (10 or 12 will do, about 2 inches deep). Place spaghetti squash in microwave and cook on high heat for about 20 minutes. To test doneness, gently squeeze with a gloved hand. If the squash gives, then it's done. If not, cook at 5-minute intervals until soft enough to give when squeezed. When done, place on cutting board and cut in half lengthwise, let stand to cool. Pound veal cutlets thin and place in egg wash, coat with ground pork rinds, and pan-fry both sides in medium hot olive oil. Put a couple of tablespoons of your favorite low-SUGAR tomato sauce on top of the cutlet along with a handful of shredded mozzarella cheese, and cover. With a fork, remove the seeds from the spaghetti squash and discard. Now, using the fork, start pulling out the squash meat onto a plate. Notice how the meat looks like strands of angel hair pasta. Salt & pepper the squash and toss with Romano or Parmesan cheese. Once the squash is "dressed," transfer portions to dinner plates.

Remove cutlets from oven and plate.

TIP—You can substitute a nice piece of thin fish, turkey, chicken cutlet, or eggplant for the veal. You can substitute Tofu Shirataki Pasta for the spaghetti squash.

Baked Shrimp with Crabmeat Stuffing

INGREDIENTS
Lump crabmeat
Shrimp
Egg
Chopped onion
Chopped green bell pepper
Shredded cheddar cheese
Salt & pepper to taste
Green salad

Buy a can of pasteurized lump crabmeat from your grocer's seafood dept. In a mixing bowl, combine 1 cup of crab, 1 egg, ¼ cup chopped onion, ¼ cup chopped green pepper, and ¼ cup shredded cheddar cheese. Use larger shrimp—size 16/20 minimum. Peel shrimp, leaving the little tail end on. Using a sharp knife, butterfly shrimp on the inside curve, opening shrimp for stuffing. Place shrimp in well buttered baking dish side by side with the tails facing up. Stuff each shrimp with a heaping teaspoon of stuffing, salt & pepper shrimp and bake in a preheated oven at 425°F for 10–12 minutes, or until shrimp is cooked through. Serve with a green salad.

COOKING TIP—Cook this recipe in individual baking dishes.

Triple Crown Baked Fish with Crabmeat Stuffing

INGREDIENTS
Lump crabmeat
Grouper filet (or other white fish)
Salmon filet
Egg
Chopped onion
Chopped green bell pepper
Shredded cheddar cheese
Salt & pepper to taste
Paprika
Butter
Capers
Lemon juice
Splenda or stevia
Green salad

Make your crabmeat stuffing as follows: Buy a can of pasteurized lump crabmeat from your grocer's seafood dept. In a mixing bowl, combine 1 cup of crab, 1 egg, ¼ cup chopped onion, ¼ cup chopped green pepper, and ¼ cup shredded cheddar cheese. Set aside. Cut a white fish filet (I prefer grouper) into 2 thinner pieces. Cut a salmon fish filet into 2 thinner pieces. Place a piece of white fish in the bottom of a well buttered baking dish, layer in crabmeat stuffing, and top with a piece of salmon. Place butter tabs on top of fish along with salt, pepper, and paprika. Repeat for second plate and bake for 20 to 25 minutes, or until fish is cooked through. Top with sweet lemon caper sauce. Spoon the sauce over the fish when served. Serve with a green salad on the side.

Sauce—Melt a half stick of butter in the microwave. To the melted butter, add 1 tablespoon of capers, 1 teaspoon of Splenda or stevia, and 1 tablespoon of lemon juice. Spoon the sauce over the fish when served. Serve with a green salad on the side.

COOKING TIP—Cook this recipe in individual baking dishes.

Salisbury Steak with Onions and Mushrooms

INGREDIENTS
Olive oil
Ground beef
Chopped onion
Heinz Home Style Turkey Gravy
Mushrooms
Cauliflower
Butter
Mayonnaise
Salt & pepper to taste

Make 4 nice sized hamburger patties and pan-fry in skillet on stove. While the burgers are cooking, toss in ½ cup rough chopped onion and ½ cup sliced mushrooms. When you turn the burgers over, pour in a jar of Heinz HomeStyle Turkey Gravy. Cover and simmer 8 minutes. Serve with cauliflower "mashed potatoes" (recipe below).

Cauliflower "Mashed Potatoes"—Prepare "mashed potatoes" by steaming a head of cauliflower in a couple of inches of water until fork tender. Drain cauliflower and place into food processor with a chopping blade. Add 2 tablespoons of your favorite mayonnaise, 1 tablespoon of Benecol spread or butter, and salt & pepper. Process until smooth.

Black and Blue Wasabi Tuna
with Spinach Salad

INGREDIENTS
Fresh tuna steaks
Olive oil
Sesame seeds
Wasabi paste
Fresh spinach
Rough chopped scallions
Rough chopped walnuts

Wasabi dressing

Buy 2 nice yellowfin or blackfin tuna steaks from your local grocer or fishmonger. Preheat 2 tablespoons of olive oil on high heat in skillet. Coat both sides of fish heavily with sesame seeds (I prefer black). Cook the fish in the hot oil no more than 12 seconds per side, and plate immediately. Fish should be very pink inside when sliced. Serve with wasabi paste on plate and a side of fresh spinach salad with wasabi dressing. I like the Tsunami brand wasabi products available in many grocers' seafood departments and at **www.afcsushi.com.**

Fresh Spinach Salad—Clean spinach and pat dry. In a mixing bowl combine spinach with rough chopped walnuts and rough chopped scallions.

Garlic Crabs and Shrimp Feast
(4 servings)

INGREDIENTS
Live blue crabs
Large shrimp
Olive oil
Diced garlic
Italian seasoning
Veggie tray
Low-sugar salad dressing (for dips)

Buy a dozen live blue crabs and 1½ pounds of shrimp from your local fishmonger. Refrigerate the blue crabs for at least 4 hours to put the crabs in a hibernation state. Take the crabs out of cold storage one by one and pop the backs off the crabs, cleaning out the guts and lungs as you go along. Preheat ¼ cup of olive oil on med/high heat. To the cold oil, add 1 whole head of garlic cloves, diced, and 2 tablespoons of Italian seasoning. When oil comes to heat, fry both sides of crabs until pink. Cook shrimp the same way until pink. Spread 4 or 5 layers of newspaper in the middle of your table, covering the entire area, and dump all the seafood in the middle. DIG IN! When done, simply roll up all the newspaper with the shells and discard. Serve with a veggie tray and salad dressing dips.

Gumbo Filet

INGREDIENTS
Boneless chicken breast
Large shrimp
Fish
Hillshire Farm Light Smoked Sausage
Chopped celery
Chopped onion
Chopped bell pepper
Crushed garlic
Okra
Cajun Land Cajun seasoning
Olive oil
Chicken stock
File powder
GG Bran CrispBread
Green salad

Heat 2 tablespoons of olive oil in the bottom of a stew pot. Brown 1 cup of 1-inch cubed chicken breast, 1 link of Hillshire Farm Light Smoked Sausage, cut into slices, ½ cup of chopped celery, ½ cup chopped onion, 3 crushed garlic cloves, and ½ cup of chopped green pepper. Once browned, pour in 5–6 cups of chicken stock (canned, no SUGAR). Bring to a boil and add 1 tablespoon Cajun Land Cajun seasoning and 1 cup of sliced okra (thawed out from freezer is OK). Reduce heat to low, simmer for 20 minutes. Add 10–12 shrimp and ½ cup of cubed fish to pot, cover and simmer another 10 minutes. Just prior to serving, sprinkle 1 teaspoon of file powder (ground sassafras) on top of stew pot and gently mix in. Serve with GG Bran CrispBread and green salad.

TIP—Freezes well for quick soup-and-salad lunch.

Pork Chops Marsala

INGREDIENTS
Pork chops
Marsala cooking wine
Whole mushrooms
Sliced yellow onion
Butter
Olive oil
Cauliflower
Butter
Mayonnaise
Salt & pepper to taste

Preheat 1 tablespoon of olive oil in a skillet over med/high heat. While the pan is heating, marinate 1 cup of whole mushrooms in 1/3 cup of Marsala cooking wine. Salt and pepper both sides of 2 1-inch-thick pork chops. Place chops in skillet and brown one side. Flip the chops over and wait 60 seconds, then pour in the mushrooms and ½ cup of thinly sliced yellow onion. Cover pan and reduce heat to med/low. Cook for 15 minutes. Remove chops and vegetables from pan, leaving the remaining liquid in pan. Plate the chops topped with vegetables and set aside. Raise heat to med/high and add 1 tablespoon of butter and ¼ cup Marsala cooking wine to pan. Reduce liquid to creamy texture and drizzle over plated chops. Serve with cauliflower "mashed potatoes" (recipe at right).

Cauliflower "Mashed Potatoes"—Prepare "mashed potatoes" by steaming a head of cauliflower in a couple of inches of water until fork tender. Drain cauliflower and place into food processor with a chopping blade. Add 2 tablespoons of your favorite mayonnaise, 1 tablespoon of Benecol spread or butter, and salt & pepper. Process until smooth.

DESSERTS

Baked Brie on Apple Slices

INGREDIENTS
Sliced apples
Brie cheese

This is one of the few times I'll use apples in a recipe; however, you can control the portions very easily. Choose a nice crisp apple like a Rome, Mac or a Granny Smith, and cut the slices very thin. Cut a big X in the top of a 4 oz wheel of Brie cheese and place into a buttered baking dish. Bake in 350°F oven until brown and bubbly, around 6 minutes. Serve on dinner plate surrounded with apple slices. Limit yourself to ¼ apple (4 carbs).

Beanit Butter Walnut Cookies

INGREDIENTS
Carb Not Beanit Butter
Eggs
Chopped walnuts
Log Cabin Sugar Free Syrup

Preheat oven to 400°F. Using Carb Not Beanit Butter (available at **www.dixiediner.com**), mix 2 eggs, ¼ cup Log Cabin Sugar Free Syrup, and ¼ cup of finely chopped walnuts to 1 15 oz jar in mixer. Roll between palms into 1-inch balls. Place another ¼ cup of finely chopped walnuts on a plate and roll the balls in additional finely chopped walnuts to coat all sides, place on cookie sheet.

Flatten down cookies with fork to about ¼-inch thick and bake for 12 minutes. Let cool and store in freezer. These are not a very sweet cookie. Wonderful with coffee, and there is a minuscule carb count from the walnuts. They are best eaten directly from the freezer.

Berry Berry Jell-O with Reddi-wip Topping

INGREDIENTS
Raspberry sugar-free Jell-O
Fresh strawberries
Fresh raspberries
Fresh blackberries
Reddi-wip topping

Make raspberry SUGAR-free Jell-O per the box instructions. Replace cold water with ice for faster set, place in fridge. Clean and chop a few strawberries, add whole raspberries and blackberries to strawberry bowl, and refrigerate. When Jell-O starts to thicken, but before set, mix in berries. Let Jell-O come to full set. Serve with Reddi-wip topping.

Berry Berry Mousse

Prepare recipe as above. When Jell-O is thick but not set, fold in an equal amount of whipped cream with the fruit. Mix gently and place in the fridge to set. Serve with whipped cream topping.

WEB-FEATURE RECIPE!—Instructional video at http://www.fattoskinny.com Click the Recipes button.

Ice Cream Cake

INGREDIENTS
TastyKake Sensables
Bryers CarbSmart low-carb ice cream
Reddi-wip topping

Using TastyKake Sensables, cut cakes in half lengthwise and place down half of the cakes as the first layer on dessert dish. Spread Bryers CarbSmart low-carb ice cream layer onto cake and top with other cake half. Top with Reddi-wip and serve.

Chocolate Dipped Strawberries

INGREDIENTS
Fresh strawberries
Sugar-free chocolate

Melt SUGAR-free chocolate in double boiler until creamy. Individually dip each whole strawberry ¾ up the berry, set on wax paper to cool.

TIP—Use cold berries to decrease chocolate set time, and make extra. They refrigerate well.

Mango Jell-O

INGREDIENTS
Peach sugar-free Jell-O
Minute Maid Light Mango Tropical Juice
Reddi-wip topping

Make packaged peach-flavored Jell-O per instructions. Replace cold water added with Minute Maid Light Mango Tropical (1g carb per can), available at your local grocer. Serve with Reddi-wip.

Strawberry Shortcake Crepes

INGREDIENTS
Eggs
New Hope Mills Low Carb Sugar Free Pancake & Waffle Mix
Butter
Fresh strawberries
Reddi-wip topping

Crepes are very easy to make. They are simply very thin pancakes used to roll up a variety of ingredients. Preheat an 8-inch nonstick skillet over medium heat. Using a stick of butter, make sure the bottom of the pan and an inch or 2 up the sides is greased. Pour in a small amount of batter and, using the pan's handle, lift and swirl the pan to spread the batter out thinly across the entire bottom of the pan. Cover pan for 60 seconds. Crepe should be set on top and can now be gently removed from pan onto a plate. Repeat the process, stacking the crepes on top of one another and separated with paper towels until you have made all the crepes you need. Follow the filling directions below.

Batter—One tablespoon of New Hope Mills Low Carb Sugar Free Pancake & Waffle Mix, 1 egg, 1 teaspoon water. Makes 2 8-inch crepes.

Filling—Mash half the strawberries into a pulp, rough chop the other half, reserving 1 whole berry for each crepe, combine berries. In a mixing bowl, start folding in whipped topping to the strawberries until you have a nice, light, fluffy mixture. Begin with twice the whipped topping to berries and add extra if necessary—do not "overwork" mixture. Place a generous amount of filling into each crepe and gently roll up. Top each crepe with a dollop of filling and a whole berry.

TIP—Blackberries or raspberries can be substitutes.

Blackberry Sorbet

INGREDIENTS
Fresh blackberries
Breyers CarbSmart low-carb ice cream
Reddi-wip topping

Mash enough ripe blackberries to measure 2 tablespoons per cup of ice cream. Using Breyers CarbSmart brand vanilla ice cream, work berries into ice cream with a fork until fully incorporated and smooth. Top with Reddi-wip and a whole berry.

TIP—Strawberries or raspberries can be substitutes.

INSTEAD OF

Many people fail on eating plans that remove their favorite foods because they hate *losing* their favorite foods. You don't have to go without; you simply need to *replace*. Use the **instead of** list below and experience some of your favorite foods with a little different flavor.

Instead of PASTA, substitute with spaghetti squash, julienned zucchini, or Tofu Shirataki Pasta.

Instead of LASAGNA NOODLES, substitute with lengthwise, thin slices of zucchini.

Instead of MASHED POTATOES, substitute with a head of steamed cauliflower, 1 tablespoon of mayonnaise, and 1 tablespoon of butter in the food processor. Process until smooth, add extra mayo if needed, and salt & pepper to taste.

Instead of FRIED POTATOES, substitute with pan-fried jicama. In a skillet, place small, diced jicama in an inch of lightly salted water. Boil jicama uncovered until water disappears. Add a tablespoon of olive oil and a teaspoon of butter to skillet, fry on medium heat for 6 or 7 minutes, and serve immediately. Jicama always retains a bit of a crunch.

Instead of BAKED POTATOES, substitute a chayote squash. Punch a couple of fork holes in the squash and microwave 5–8 minutes or until fork tender. Serve as a baked potato with sour cream and butter.

Instead of FRIED FOOD COATING, substitute with non-sweetened pork rinds ground fine in a food processor.

Instead of CORN STARCH GRAVY THICKENER, substitute with ThickenThin not/Starch Thickener, available at many low-carb websites.

Instead of BREAD, substitute with romaine lettuce leaves, GG Bran CrispBread, or low-carb tortillas.

Instead of FLOUR TORTILLAS, substitute with La Tortilla Factory tortillas.

Instead of SUGAR SODA, substitute with SUGAR-free soda.

Instead of SUGAR, substitute with stevia sweetener.

Instead of PIZZA, use low-carb tortillas and make a personal pizza loaded with cheese, meats, and veggies from the list.

Your personal *instead of* list will grow as you play around with your ingredients, as will your recipes. Don't be afraid to try new ideas as they present themselves to you. I look forward to reading YOUR recipes. Send to: **dougvarrieur@fattoskinny.com.**

"I HATE COOKING! WHAT DO I DO?"

Hate to cook? Don't worry—I have you covered! Let's take a look at the reality of what you'll need to do. Most of the time, eating low-SUGAR is more about taking food *off* your plate vs. what goes *on* your plate. And don't worry about where your snack trays will come from. Most supermarkets and delis have or can prepare any kind of tray you want. Veggie trays, meat trays, cheese trays, and chicken wing trays are all very common.

It's time to learn what to take *off* the plate. Due to your SUGAR sensitivity, you simply can't eat some of the items on the plate. Ask your waitstaff not to include them on your plate, and I'm certain they will oblige your needs.

BREAKFAST

The following items, written in **bold italic**, contain SUGAR and should be avoided on this eating plan: ***bagels, bread, English muffins, fried potatoes, grits, hash browns, muffins, pancakes***. Also avoid all table SUGAR and syrups. Sweeten your coffee, if you wish, with artificial sweetener, and ask your waitstaff for a small server of cream from the kitchen to lighten it. Diet soda, brewed teas, and water with a squeeze of lemon are also available.

LUNCH

"What About Fast Food?"

Many fast food restaurants also include salads on their menus. Order a couple of burgers and a green salad, throw away the *bun*, and break up the burgers on top of your salad. Top with a low-SUGAR dressing. Hidden Valley Ranch is usually available. Carry a low-carb tortilla with you from home and use it as a wrap to replace the bun, if you wish.

"What About Chinese?"

Most Chinese restaurants use cornstarch and savory sauces in their dishes. One tablespoon of *cornstarch* has about 7 grams of carbs, and the *sauces* are loaded with salt and...??? The safe bet is to order any of the meat or seafood/vegetable combinations *WITHOUT ANY SAUCES*. Simply tell the wait staff that you are sensitive to SUGAR and you simply want your meal stir-fried in the wok with nothing added. Ask for butter on the side, and tab the meal with butter. Soy sauce is about ½ gram carbs per teaspoon, and the hot mustard on the table is usually carb-free. Stay away from all the *sweet and sour dishes*, all *deep fried coatings*, *all sauces*, the *sweet sauce* on the table, and yes...the *fortune cookie*. You can open it though... the fortune inside will say, "A new and leaner you is just around the corner." ☺ Then, throw the *cookie* away; it's loaded with SUGAR.

"What About Mexican?"

Mexican is pretty limited. *Tortillas, both flour and corn* are a mainstay, so are *refried beans* and *corn chips* with salsa. Your safe bet is to order chicken or beef fajitas and don't eat the *tortillas*. Usually the side plate includes lettuce, cheddar cheese, sour cream, and *refried beans*. Avoid the *refried beans* as well.

"What About Italian?"

Italian is also limited. Once again, the menu will be loaded with SUGAR. It will be in the form of *pasta* and *bread*. Your best bet is to order meatballs in sauce topped with cheese and melted in the oven, a green salad, and whatever green vegetable of the day they offer (other than peas). You can also ask for any meat, fish, or poultry available on the menu to be pan-fried for you in olive oil without any coatings or sauces. Ask for any sauces to be delivered on the side.

DINNER

Any seafood or steakhouse is a great choice. One of my favorites is Outback Steakhouse. They always have a wide selection that fits this low-SUGAR eating plan. Always stick with meats, seafood, and green vegetables, sauce free. Never include the *potato* or the *bread* in your meal. Check out **www.outback.com**.

By now you should be getting pretty comfortable with where the SUGAR is coming from in restaurants.

The **main culprits to avoid** are the following:

rice
grits
pasta
sauces
breads
potatoes
pancakes
fry coatings
table chips and snacks
high-SUGAR vegetables
and salad dressings

The foods to order are the same ones on your ingredient list in this book. Take it with you and be vocal with your waitstaff about your needs. This is your body, and you're addicted to SUGAR. Obviously, eating out will not be a problem for you. After a while, all of this information will become second nature to you and you'll SEE the SUGAR in all the foods presented to you through your lifetime. You'll become SKINNY and happier with your body. You'll wonder why no one in school ever taught you the simplicity of staying thin. You'll wonder why so many people spend so much money on diets and diet programs that simply do not work. You'll become vocal and feel the need, as I do, to share your miracle with other people who are obviously struggling with their own **FAT** issues.

When you feel that urge, tell them about your new-found book, **FAT TO SKINNY Fast and Easy!**, and smile as they walk away wondering if maybe, just maybe, there is hope for them, too!

REACHING OPTIMUM WEIGHT

First, a word for the ladies. Hello, ladies. I'm excited for you. I know you've decided to take the steps outlined in this book to eat yourself back into good health and a size…??? I'm sure you've noticed that throughout the book, I've kept size to *your* discretion. How much you *should* weigh is entirely relative to your body size, breast size, and age. Don't let front-page, airbrushed models intimidate you. There is no rule that says you need to weigh 115 pounds and be a size 4! Your goal should be to get your blood sugar levels back into check and let your body find its *optimum weight*. Be patient. The sad truth is you'll lose **FAT** more slowly than will your male counterparts. If you and a guy are starting this quest together, he will most likely beat you to the finish line, so don't bet him! It can be frustrating to a woman to have her guy dropping weight faster than she is. Don't let it bother you; just stay the course and charge forward. You didn't gain all this **FAT** overnight, and you won't lose it overnight.

Now, including the guys: Let's talk about the steps to *optimum weight*. It begins with *plateaus*. If your weight stays the same for more than 3 weeks, you've reached a *plateau*. Don't fret! Plateaus are a good thing. At this point, your body is efficiently burning all the food you're eating based on your normal activity level. You're making progress! Now it's time to evaluate where you are, where you want to go, and what to do about it. If you're happy with your size, then you have reached your optimum weight. Keep eating the same, keep your activity level the same, and your size will stay the same. If you're unhappy with your size, then it's time to *tweak*. You have 3 choices:

1- **Keep your food intake the same and increase your activity level.**

2- **Change your food intake and leave your activity level the same.**

3- **Change your food intake and increase your activity level.**

You already know how to increase your activity level, so let's talk about your food. The first thing to look at is what you're eating. Start by removing ALL SUGAR alcohols and artificial sweeteners from your intake. Remove ALL packaged foods, such as pancake mixes and tortillas. Stick only to protein and a measured amount of veggies from the veggie list. The second thing to look at is the *amount* of food you're eating. Are your portions too large? Your body is changing as your **FAT** is burning; it's adjusting to your new low-SUGAR eating plan and is different from what it was when we did our first "what is hungry?" experiment. It's time to do our experiment again. Use the next 3 days to get to know your new metabolism. Eat only when you are certain you're eating for the right reasons, *and* only eat as much food as you need to satisfy that natural hunger. In most cases, men and woman find their answer is in their food. SUGAR in condiments, portion control, and eating for the wrong reasons are usually the culprits. Adding additional activity without recognizing the other factors will only bring temporary relief, so start with the food.

AUTHOR'S PERSONAL BLOOD PROFILE

Do you remember the criticism I mentioned to you that I was receiving from friends about my eating plan? I would like to discuss with you a criticism that you're bound to hear from friends and family. My blood profile was brought into question on more than one occasion. People, including my own doctor, found it hard to believe that I could eat a diet so high in proteins and fats without a negative impact on my blood. So to keep a solid record and to be certain of my course of action, I had my blood profile taken at over 215 pounds and then again at 165 pounds. Here are the results:

BEFORE

Triglycerides	400
HDL Cholesterol	45
LDL Cholesterol	199
CHOL/HDLC Ratio	5.07
Total Cholesterol	**257**

AFTER

Triglycerides	70
HDL Cholesterol	50
LDL Cholesterol	145
CHOL/HDLC Ratio	4.2
Total Cholesterol	**209**

As you can clearly see, my *triglycerides* dropped an amazing 330 points. What can cause high triglycerides? Triglyceride levels usually increase as your weight increases. Excess calories, especially from SUGAR and alcohol, are one of the causes of high triglycerides. Alcohol increases your liver's production of triglycerides and reduces the amount of **FAT** cleared from your blood. Triglyceride testing measures the amount of triglycerides in your blood. Triglycerides are the body's storage form for **FAT**. Most triglycerides are found in *adipose* (**FAT**) tissue. Some triglycerides circulate in the blood to provide fuel for muscle function. Extra triglycerides end up in storage in *adipose* (**FAT**) tissue. Triglycerides are the form of **FAT** found in various lipoproteins in the bloodstream. High levels of triglycerides are usually a sign of high levels of insulin. It was a great relief to see them drop so dramatically. Not only did my body get SKINNY, but my blood got SKINNY, as well!

To control cholesterol, I have added *plant sterols* to my daily diet. Plant sterols have been proven to reduce and control cholesterol. In tablet form, they are available in the brand CholestOff available over the counter at Walmart. They are also available in the vegetable oil spread, Benecol, also available at Walmart.

My HDL cholesterol (the good one) increased 5 points.

LDL cholesterol is the bad cholesterol and should

be watched carefully by all of us. My personal LDL cholesterol dropped 54 points as a direct result of adding CholestOff and Benecol to my daily intake of supplements. The 54-point drop occurred in only 90 days! You can locate info on CholestOff and Benecol at the following web sites:

www.cholestoff.com
www.benecol.com

Being heavy most of my life and maintaining high cholesterol levels took its toll on my body, and at 50 years old I have my share of plaque in my arteries. My doctors have furthered my quest to reduce my total cholesterol by prescribing a *statin* drug called Lipitor. I'm told by my doctors that this particular *statin* drug has a dual effect: Not only will it reduce my total cholesterol, but it also provides an anti-inflammatory function designed to keep the existing plaque from become inflamed within my arteries (which would cause reduced blood flow). I am also very careful to avoid all trans fats, and I keep saturated fats to a minimum by choosing the leanest cuts of meat, watching animal meat portions, whole egg and cheese portions, and including fish and soy protein in my diet a couple times per week.

If you're heavy and have been for some length of time, I recommend you consult with your doctors to discuss your personal blood profile. Your doctor may recommend a nuclear stress test, which I highly recommend. This non-invasive test is a simple way for your doctor to take a peek inside your heart. This will give your doctor—and you—an opportunity to see if you have any impending blockages that need addressing *before* you experience a lapse in heart function. I also take a multivitamin and a B12 vitamin every day.

The long and the short of it is as simple as the blood results on the reports:

Remove SUGAR from your life, and you will become healthier.

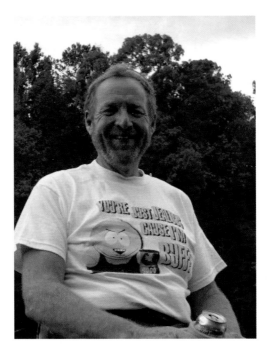

EPILOGUE

Thank you for taking the time to allow me to share my story with you. I wrote **FAT TO SKINNY Fast and Easy!** because I knew I could help people of all ages. There's simply no reason for anyone to go through life as a fAT person if they know the secrets. With the rising obesity problem our nation is facing, children's education became an important part of my mission. I tried to write this book to be easily understood by all ages, and if you have children I urge you to have them read it. Starting your kids eating right when they are young will be a lifelong gift they will appreciate as they get older. Before you start your program, take a BEFORE photo of yourself and email it to me. I'll be rooting for you and will look forward to your AFTER photo showing your success. I would like to hear from you and learn how the information contained in this book has helped to change your life. Please feel free to contact me by email:

dougvarrieur@fattoskinny.com

About the Author

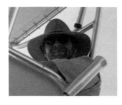

Doug Varrieur

Entrepreneur, businessman, father, stepfather, husband, ex-husband, son, stepson, partner, ex-partner, writer, and philosopher

Here are some interesting facts about the author. When Doug wrote **FAT TO SKINNY Fast and Easy!**, he was 50 years young. He had battled weight gain his entire life until he found the secrets. Being **FAT** never held him back, and over the past 27 years he built and sold 3 successful companies and worked extensively as a business consultant. The only challenge Doug couldn't succeed at over the years was weight control. He put all of his effort and time into finding the secrets to **FAT** loss and good health. He succeeded, quickly and easily losing over 100 pounds with his own methods. Next came Sherri's amazing 70-pound **FAT** loss, all without diets, surgery, drugs, or exercise. Doug found the SECRET! **FAT TO SKINNY Fast and Easy!** was written because he wanted to share his secrets with the world. Over 5 years after this amazing weight loss, Doug and Sherri, his beautiful wife of 8 years, continue to enjoy being thin and healthy. They concentrate on living a well-balanced and happy life.